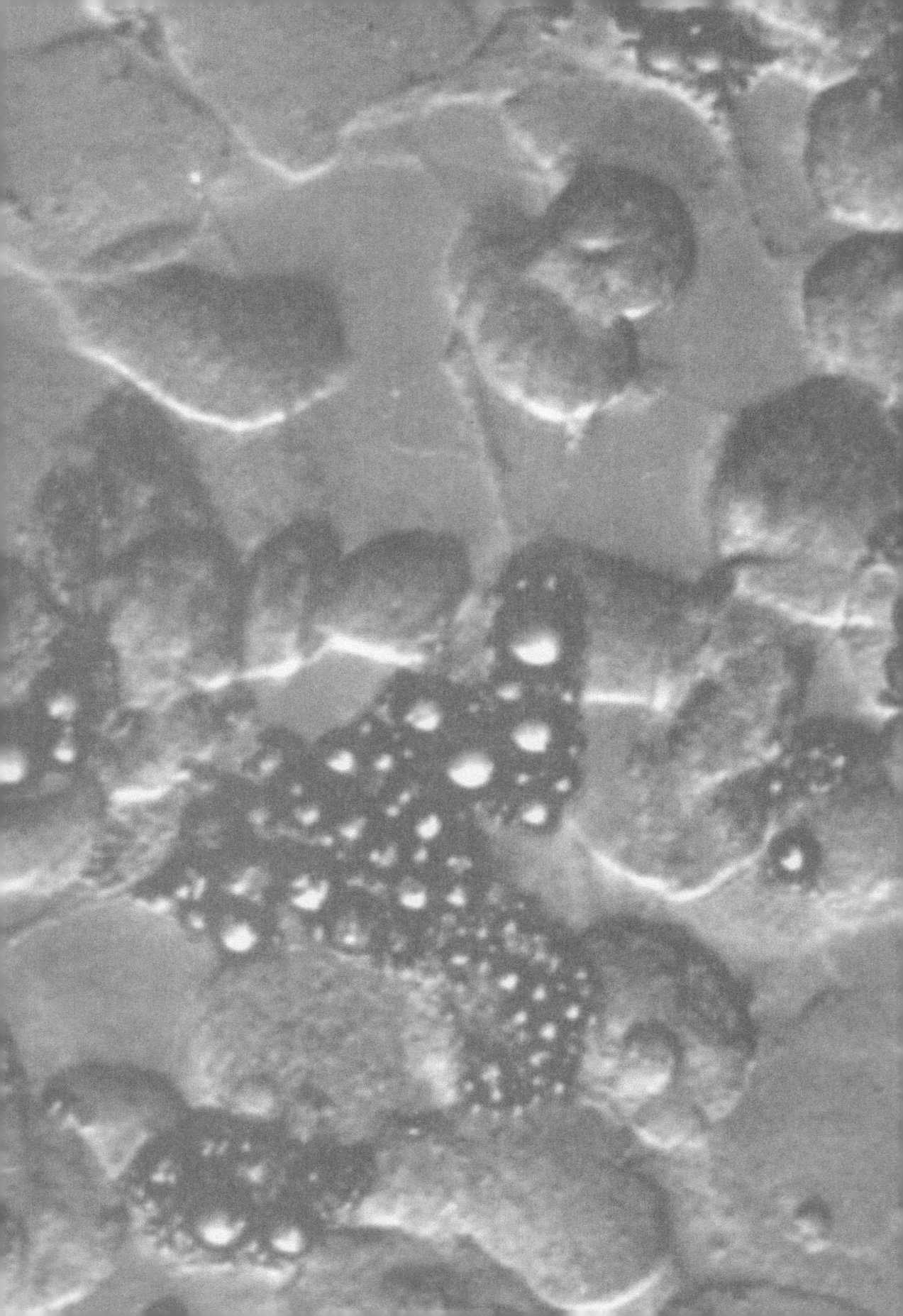

Effect of IL-10 and anti-TGF beta
antibodies on the morphology of
bone marrow stromal culture
from
Interleukin-10
by
Jan E. de Vries and
René de Waal Malefyt
©RG Landes Co. 1995

MOLECULAR
BIOLOGY
INTELLIGENCE
UNIT

WILMS TUMOR: CLINICAL AND MOLECULAR CHARACTERIZATION

Max J. Coppes, M.D., Ph.D.

Tom Baker Cancer Centre and University of Calgary
Calgary, Alberta, Canada

Christine E. Campbell, Ph.D.

Bryan R.G. Williams, Ph.D.

Department of Cancer Biology Research Institute
Cleveland Clinic Foundation
Cleveland, Ohio, USA

Springer-Verlag Berlin Heidelberg GmbH

MOLECULAR BIOLOGY INTELLIGENCE UNIT

WILMS TUMOR: CLINICAL AND MOLECULAR CHARACTERIZATION

International Copyright © 1995 Springer-Verlag Berlin Heidelberg
Originally published by Springer-Verlag in 1995
Softcover reprint of the hardcover 1st edition 1995

International ISBN 978-3-662-22623-0

Library of Congress Cataloging-in-Publication Data

Coppes, Max
   Wilms Tumor: Clinical and Molecular Characterization/ Max Coppes.
      p. cm. — (Molecular biology intelligence unit)
   Includes bibliographical references and index.
   ISBN 978-3-662-22623-0   ISBN 978-3-662-22621-6 (eBook)
   DOI 10.1007/978-3-662-22621-6

   1. Nephroblastoma—Molecular aspects. I. Title. II. Series. [DNLM: 1. Nephroblastoma. 2. Kidney Neoplasms—in infancy & childhood. 3. Genes, Wilms Tumor. WJ 358C785w 1995]
   RC280.K5C67 1995
618.92'99261—dc20
DNLM/DLC   95-14340
for Library of Congress   CIP

PUBLISHER'S NOTE

R.G. Landes Company publishes five book series: *Medical Intelligence Unit, Molecular Biology Intelligence Unit, Neuroscience Intelligence Unit, Tissue Engineering Intelligence Unit* and *Biotechnology Intelligence Unit*. The authors of our books are acknowledged leaders in their fields and the topics are unique. Almost without exception, no other similar books exist on these topics.

Our goal is to publish books in important and rapidly changing areas of medicine for sophisticated researchers and clinicians. To achieve this goal, we have accelerated our publishing program to conform to the fast pace in which information grows in biomedical science. Most of our books are published within 90 to 120 days of receipt of the manuscript. We would like to thank our readers for their continuing interest and welcome any comments or suggestions they may have for future books.

Deborah Muir Molsberry
Publications Director
R.G. Landes Company

CONTENTS

PREFACE

Wilms tumor is a common pediatric neoplasm of the kidney which has been considered a paradigm for understanding the etiology of embryonal tumors. Although the prognosis for patients diagnosed with this childhood cancer is excellent overall, there is a clear need to improve our ability to distinguish patients requiring intensive therapy, with its subsequent risks of serious side effects, from those who will respond successfully to less radical treatments.

The study of Wilms tumor has been considerably advanced by the identification and cloning by our group and others of a Wilms tumor suppressor gene, *WT1* that maps to human chromosome 11p13. Mutations in this gene have been unequivocally shown to underlie the development of certain Wilms tumors. In addition, however, *WT1* mutations have also been demonstrated to play a role in other disorders, most notably in a rare syndrome of pseudohermaphroditism, glomerulopathy and Wilms tumor (Denys-Drash syndrome).

Since the identification of *WT1*, it has become increasingly clear that Wilms tumor is a genetically heterogeneous disease involving other loci and additional tumor suppressor genes. This book integrates what is currently known about the clinical presentation and treatment of Wilms tumors, the histopathology of pediatric kidney neoplasms, syndromes associated with Wilms tumor and the molecular genetic basis of the disease. The latter include the cloning and characterization of the *WT1* locus and patterns of expression and cellular function of the WT1 protein. The naturally occurring mutations that have thus far been described are summarized. Finally, we discuss other loci implicated in Wilms tumor, i.e. *WIT1* on chromosome 11p13, the putative Wilms tumor suppressor gene *WT2* on chromosome 11p15, yet unidentified loci on chromosomes 1p and 16q, the *p53* gene on chromosome 17p and the unidentified familial Wilms tumor gene.

In addition to describing current knowledge, we speculate on areas of future research that will be important to pursue to further our understanding of this tumor.

Max J. Coppes
Christine E. Campbell
Bryan R.G. Williams

CHAPTER 1

CLINICAL PRESENTATION AND TREATMENT

INTRODUCTION

In the past two decades, there has been a considerable improvement in the understanding and management of Wilms tumor and other primary renal childhood malignancies. Wilms tumor is usually diagnosed in children under the age of six, although occasionally older children are affected. Current treatment for Wilms tumor includes surgery and chemotherapy for all patients and radiation therapy for those with advanced disease or specific adverse prognostic features. This has led to cure rates exceeding 80%,[1] permitting most affected children to reach adulthood.

Clinically, Wilms tumor has been associated with certain congenital defects, most notably aniridia (the absence of the iris) and genitourinary malformations. Also, it sometimes occurs in children with growth altering syndromes, for example hemihypertrophy or Beckwith-Wiedemann syndrome (BWS). Children with any of the above-mentioned congenital disorders are at increased risk of developing Wilms tumor and consequently need to be screened,[2,3] although the means by which these children need to be followed still remains to be determined. However, as we will describe, the association of Wilms tumor with certain congenital anomalies has played a crucial role in identifying genetic loci involved in this malignancy.

The first chapter of this book will outline some of the notable clinical features of Wilms tumor and its treatment. In addition,

Wilms Tumor: Clinical and Molecular Characterization, by Max J. Coppes, Christine E. Campbell, and Bryan R.G. Williams. © 1995 R.G. Landes Company.

we will describe the most important recognizable patterns of malformation associated with this childhood cancer.

EPIDEMIOLOGY

Epidemiologic studies suggest that genetic factors are important in the etiology of Wilms tumor. First, the occurrence of the disease is remarkably constant among peoples in scattered parts of the world who have different environments and lifestyles. If anything, the variation seems more closely associated with race than geography.[4] The approximate 3- to 4-fold ratio in maximum to minimum rate worldwide (Table 1.1) is substantially less than the ratios of 10-20 typically observed for adult epithelial cancers in which environmental factors are known to play a pivotal role.[4] A second observation, that suggests an important role for genetic rather than epidemiologic factors in Wilms tumorigenesis, is the demonstrated association of Wilms tumor with certain congenital anomalies such as aniridia and hemihypertrophy (see later).

INCIDENCE

Wilms tumor accounts for 6-7% of all childhood cancers in the United States. The overall annual incidence in children under 15 years of age is approximately seven cases (range 5.9 to 14.6 cases) per million.[7,8] Most Caucasian populations have age standardized rates of 6-9 cases per million person years and a cumulative incidence of slightly more than one case per 10,000 children

Table 1.1. Age standardized rates of Wilms tumor per million person years

United States, African Americans	10.9
Nigeria	10.3
Sweden	9.2
Italy	7.5
Brazil	7.2
Canada	7.2
United States, Caucasians	7.1
Israel	6.8
Kuwait	3.8
Japan	3.2
China	2.5

Reproduced from Stiller and Parkin,[5] Breslow,[4] and Coppes.[6]

from birth to age 15 years.[4] Rates in several East Asian populations are in the range of 3-4 per million person years, while those in Black populations in the United States and in some African countries exceed 10 per million per year.[4] The fact that such variations exist more closely associated with race than geography suggests that environmental risk factors likely play a minor etiologic role, certainly in comparison with adult epithelial cancers.[4]

Most registries worldwide report a sex ratio close to one,[8] although in North America the rate for girls is 22% higher than for boys.[4] The significance of this observation remains to be determined and further data from incidence registers are required in order to resolve the issue of a possible sex difference in Wilms tumor.

AGE AT PRESENTATION

Wilms tumor is primarily a disease of childhood and typically affects young children. The overall median age is 3.5 years.[1] Occasionally older children and even adults[9] can be affected. Age at diagnosis according to ethnicity has revealed that Blacks are diagnosed at slightly older ages (median 41 months) and Asians at somewhat younger ages (median 30 months) compared to Caucasians (median 36 months).[4] The significance of this observation has yet to be established.

Somewhat surprisingly, a notable difference has been found in median age at diagnosis in relation to sex. Females are on average six months older at diagnosis than male patients.[4,10,11] The difference is significant for patients with unilateral Wilms tumor. Although the age at diagnosis in bilateral Wilms tumor also differs between the two sexes, it does not reach statistical significance, probably because of small numbers. The implications of these observations with regard to Wilms tumorigenesis remain unclear.

Most children present with a unilateral tumor, but approximately 5-10% of children are affected with bilateral disease.[12] Children with bilateral disease at presentation (synchronous bilateral Wilms tumor) are diagnosed, on average, a full year before those with unilateral (either unicentric or multicentric) disease.[10,11] Those initially presenting with unilateral Wilms tumor but subsequently developing bilateral disease (asynchronous or metachronous bilateral Wilms tumor) are considerably younger at first presentation than those presenting with bilateral disease at onset (synchronous bilateral Wilms tumor).[12,13] Also, patients with characteristic genitourinary abnormalities, aniridia or BWS are significantly younger at diagnosis than are those without the same congenital anomalies; those with hemihypertrophy, however, are not.[4] Patients with intralobar nephrogenic rests (ILNRs, see chapter 2) are substantially younger at diagnosis than those with perilobar nephrogenic rests (PLNRs, see chapter 2) or with neither precursor lesions. As discussed in chapter 3, some of these observations have helped to formulate the two-hit hypothesis for the development of this tumor. Somewhat surprisingly, investigators have failed to demonstrate younger age at diagnosis for the small group of patients with familial Wilms tumor. This observation is curious since a suspected age difference was used as evidence in support of the two-stage mutational model for the origin of Wilms tumor.[14]

ENVIRONMENTAL RISK FACTORS

Cancer epidemiologists have attempted to correlate the occurrence of Wilms tumor with parental environmental exposures that could affect the germ cells or the developing fetus. Unfortunately, none of the studies thus far reported have analyzed more than 200 cases of Wilms tumor. Moreover, virtually all studies have attempted to link those cases with a large number of different occupational and exposure categories. As a consequence, the data generated are inconclusive: some studies suggest an association with paternal exposure to hydrocarbons or lead, others are unable to confirm these observations.[4] Similarly, investigations into whether maternal exposures prior to conception or during the pregnancy are associated with the development of Wilms tumor, have resulted in inconsistent findings. No particular exposures have been identified as having a statistically significant association with the development of Wilms tumor. Individual studies have found links with consumption of coffee or tea, smoking cigarettes, use of oral contraceptives or other hormones, use of hair dyes, hypertension, vaginal infection during the pregnancy, or use of penthrane anesthesia.[15,16] However, none of these have been consistently replicated.[4] Consequently, while there remains a possibility that parental exposures to environmental carcinogens could play an etiologic factor in the development of Wilms tumor, additional studies are required. Once the genetic factors that underlie Wilms tumorigenesis have been identified, the analysis of environmental factors associated with the development of this tumor may prove of great value in elucidating the mechanisms that lead to the genetic defects.

CLINICAL PRESENTATION

The most common initial clinical manifestation of Wilms tumor is the presence of an asymptomatic abdominal mass, often found unintentionally by either parents or relatives, or by a physician in the course of a routine physical examination. When first discovered most Wilms tumors are quite large (Fig. 1.1). Three possible factors might contribute to this. First, retroperitoneal masses can grow undisturbed by strict anatomical boundaries. Second, functional defects in paired organs with a good functional reserve are unlikely to be detected in an early phase and third, most young children are unable to verbalize their complaints adequately.

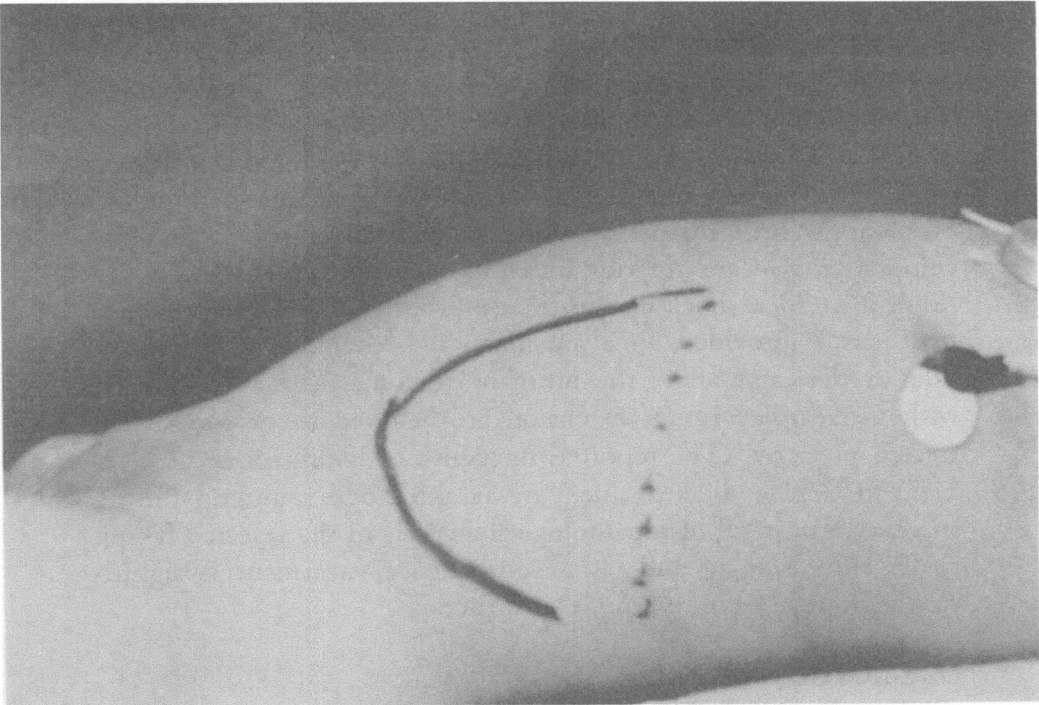

Fig. 1.1. Left-sided Wilms tumor prior to surgical removal

Signs and symptoms in addition to the presence of an abdominal mass include abdominal pain, hematuria, either gross or microscopic, fever of unknown origin, anorexia, vomiting and malaise.[1] Each of these symptoms are found in 5-30% of cases. Additional symptoms mainly arise through tumor invasion or compression of adjacent or more remote organs.

A distinct group of symptoms suggests that Wilms tumor may produce bioactive substances.[17] These include hypertension, present in about 25% of the cases[18] and acquired von Willebrand disease, present in <10% of children.[19] However, the documented production of some polypeptides does not manifest clinical symptoms. These include erythropoietin,[20,21] (pro) renin,[22,23] hyaluronic acid,[24] hyaluronic acid stimulating activity[25] and hyaluronidase.[26] The clinical significance of these biological markers to diagnosis or prognosis has not yet been established.

PATTERNS OF EXTENSION AND METASTASES AT DIAGNOSIS

Tumor spread usually does not lead to specific clinical manifestations, but often will be detectable by radiological studies. The most common sites of metastases at diagnosis are the lungs and the liver.[27] In addition, approximately 8% of the patients present with non-hematogeneous hepatic involvement, i.e. hepatic adhesion or invasion,[28] and another 10-15% will manifest intravenous extension.[29] In most cases, extension involves the renal vein lumen only, but extension into the vena cava inferior is not uncommon. Surprisingly little discomfort and few clinical symptoms may accompany vena cava inferior invasion, although embolization can result in sudden shock due to tricuspid obstruction. If appropriate treatment is provided, involvement of the renal vein or vena cava inferior does not affect the ultimate outcome, and even patients with intracardiac tumor extension are believed to do well when treated properly.[1] The reported incidence of lymph node involvement, 15-20%, dictates adequate lymph node sampling during surgery and careful histopathological analysis of the resected lymph nodes since staging and, as a consequence, treatment is significantly altered if positive nodes are found.

DIAGNOSTIC IMAGING

The primary goals of radiologic evaluation are: 1) to confirm that the palpated tumor indeed originates from the kidney;

2) to determine its nature; and 3) to determine its extension. This will help develop an appropriate plan of treatment. Consequently, the imaging studies selected should take into account the specific characteristics of Wilms tumor and its metastatic pattern. A computed axial tomography (CAT) scan of both abdomen (Fig. 1.2) and chest with the use of intravenous contrast usually provides most of the information needed. Nevertheless, in the majority of North American institutions, abdominal CAT scanning will be proceeded by ultrasonography, a procedure that provides valuable initial information especially on the vascular extent of an abdominal tumor. Moreover, ultrasonography has no known serious side effects. Other institutions use ultrasonography and intravenous pelography as the primary imaging techniques. The ultimate

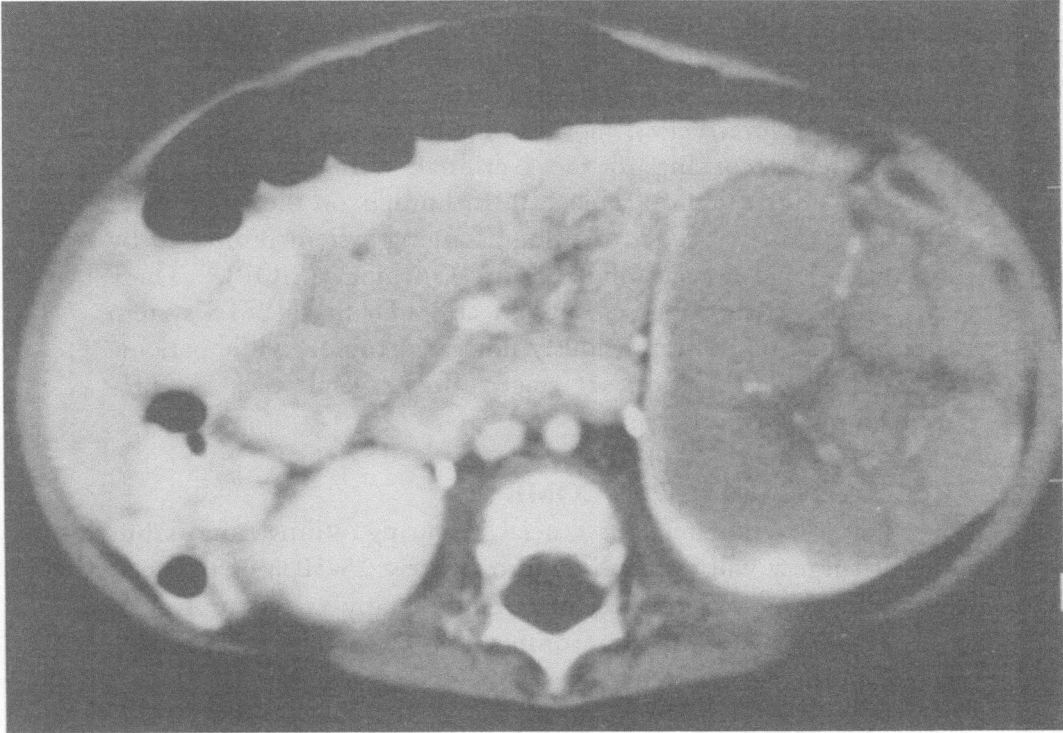

Fig. 1.2. CAT-scan image of left-sided Wilms tumor. Axial enhanced CAT-scan image of the upper abdomen demonstrating a large solid non-homogeneous exophytic mass arising from the left kidney. Note the thin rim of normal renal tissue along the medial and posterior aspect of the mass. Reprinted with permission from M.J. Coppes, Wilms tumor: From cure to understanding, Critical Reviews in Oncology and Hematology 1995; 18:179-196. Copyright © Elsevier Scientific Publishers, Ireland Ltd.

determination on the sequence of radiological examinations that should be performed is based on several factors: availability of each modality, quality of the machines used, expertise with the available modalities, undesired side effects, as well as cost interests and risks.

STAGING

Standardized tumor staging is important in allowing proper evaluation of different patient treatments. At the present time staging is primarily based on the anatomical extent of the disease. However, all patients are also classified according to histopathology, as described in chapter 2, since this has proven useful in predicting relapse and outcome.

Ideally, the TNM classification,[30] which is based on the size of the primary tumor (T), regional lymph node involvement (N), and the occurrence of distant metastases (M), should be used to classify all tumors. The TNM classification provides an objective standard staging system, enabling worldwide comparison of management results. Nevertheless, most Wilms tumors in North America are classified according to the National Wilms Tumor Study (NWTS) staging system[1] (Table 1.2). In Europe, on the other hand, children are usually classified using a staging system promoted by the International Society of Paediatric Oncology (SIOP).[31] These two staging systems are very similar, although the NWTS system is based on staging of a previously untreated tumor, while patients in the SIOP classification are staged after several weeks of prenephrectomy chemotherapy.

TREATMENT AND OUTCOME

Surgical excision remains crucial in curing Wilms tumors but by itself surgery will only cure approximately 15-30% of patients. The addition of post-nephrectomy radiotherapy raises survival to approximately 50%, while the combination of surgery, radiotherapy and chemotherapy will cure over 80% of patients.

SURGICAL MANAGEMENT

There have been no major changes to the surgical approach of Wilms tumor since its development and perfection by William Ladd.[32] The standard technique is transabdominal transperitoneal, with emphasis on the necessity for a generous incision that allows

Table 1.2. NWTS clinicopathologic staging

stage I   *Tumor limited to the kidney and completely excised*
The surface of the renal capsule is intact. The tumor was not ruptured before or during removal. There is no residual tumor apparent beyond the margins of excision.

stage II   *Tumor extends beyond the kidney, but is completely excised*
There is regional extension of the tumor (i.e., penetration through the surface of the renal capsule into the perirenal soft tissue). Vessels outside the kidney substance are infiltrated or contain tumor thrombus. The tumor may have been biopsied or there has been local spillage of tumor confined to the flank. There is no residual tumor apparent at or beyond the margins of excision.

stage III   *Residual nonhematogenous tumor confined to the abdomen*
Any of the following may occur: a) lymph nodes on biopsy are found to be involved in the hilus, the periaortic chains, or beyond; b) there has been diffuse peritoneal contamination by the tumor, such as spillage of the tumor beyond the flank before or during surgery, or tumor growth that has penetrated on the peritoneal surfaces; c) implants are found on the peritoneal surfaces; d) the tumor extends beyond the surgical margins either microscopically or grossly; e) the tumor is not completely resectable because of local infiltration into vital structures.

stage IV   *Hematogenous metastases*
Deposits beyond stage III (lung, liver, bones and brain).

stage V   *Bilateral renal involvement at diagnosis*

The clinical staging is decided by the surgeon in the operating room and is confirmed by a pathologist who also evaluates the histology. Staging is the same for tumors with favorable and with unfavorable histology. However, every patient will be characterized by a statement of both criteria (e.g., stage II/ favorable histology, or stage I unfavorable histology).[1]

thorough inspection of the intra-abdominal contents.[33] Inspection of the contralateral kidney is preferably accomplished prior to ipsilateral nephrectomy, as the total surgical and oncologic approach of the affected patient is considerably altered following demonstration of bilateral disease. Special attention should also be given to the liver and para-aortic area. Routine radical lymph node dissection, while advocated in the past, is currently not recommended. However, in order to achieve correct staging, adequate lymph node sampling should be performed.

RADIATION TREATMENT

Radiotherapy has been utilized mainly as an adjuvant to surgery. In fact it has been standard practice until recently to offer post-nephrectomy radiotherapy to all patients, usually immediately after surgical removal of the affected kidney. However, the advent of highly effective chemotherapeutic drugs has impacted on the use of radiotherapy, especially since long-term follow-up data revealed serious late side effects attributed to radiotherapy. In the past two decades, it was demonstrated that certain patients, for instance those with stage I or stage II disease and favorable histology, do not require post-nephrectomy radiotherapy when they are given adequate chemotherapy.[34-36] The goal of current protocols is to define high risk groups that need radiotherapy routinely, versus those that can be cured with surgery and chemotherapy alone. Meanwhile, the total radiation dose, if radiation therapy is required, has been reduced from approximately 4000 cGy to 1100 cGy.[37]

CHEMOTHERAPY

Three drugs have demonstrated a high efficacy in the treatment of Wilms tumor: actinomycin D (AMD), vincristine (VCR) and doxorubicin (DOX). Several additional drugs, including cyclophosphamide, ifosfamide, bleomycin, etoposide and cisplatin are under further investigation.

AMD is a chemotherapeutic agent of a group of antitumor antibiotics identified in 1940. The drug's yellow color is due to the tricyclic phenoxazone chromophore, which is linked to two short, identical cyclic polypeptides. The chromophore permits intercalation between base pairs in DNA, with a preference for guanine, while the polypeptide rings lie in the minor groove of DNA. This binding to DNA results in inhibition of RNA and subsequent protein synthesis. AMD has a potentiating effect on radiation therapy.[38] As a result, lower dosages of radiation should be given when AMD is administered concurrently. At present, AMD is one of the two chemotherapeutic drugs routinely utilized in the treatment of virtually all Wilms tumors.

VCR is an alkaloid extracted from the herb Vinca Rosea Linn. It exerts its anti-neoplastic effect by blocking cell division at metaphase. Its effectiveness as a single drug in Wilms tumor treatment was first demonstrated in 1963.[39] Together with AMD, VCR is routinely used in the treatment of all Wilms tumors.

DOX is a anthracycline antibiotic produced from the mold *Streptomyces peucetius*. DOX binds to DNA by intercalation between adjacent base pairs. Its mechanisms of action involve inhibition of DNA topoisomerase II and the inhibition of both DNA replication and DNA directed RNA synthesis. Following preliminary reports on its efficacy in advanced Wilms tumor, DOX was entered into a Phase II study in 1969.[40] Subsequently DOX was incorporated in major clinical Wilms tumor trials. However, the recent demonstration of serious cardiotoxic side effects has resulted in a re-evaluation of the routine use of this drug. Currently only patients with advanced stage disease receive this drug routinely.

SURVIVAL

Efficient multimodal treatment has decreased the incidence of local and/or distant tumor recurrence to <25%. Most relapses occur within the first two years following nephrectomy, although late recurrences have been reported. The sites most frequently affected are lungs, abdomen and liver.[27]

Treatment of cancer is associated with side effects — some occurring early, others being revealed only after many years. The excellent life expectancy in patients with Wilms tumor has resulted in the identification of previously unexpected late effects, affecting several organ systems, including the musculoskeletal, renal, cardiovascular, pulmonary and endocrine systems.[41]

The heart may be damaged by radiation therapy and several chemotherapeutic agents. A particular concern is the dosage-related cardiomyopathy caused by the anthracycline DOX.[42] The cumulative percentage of children treated with DOX for Wilms tumor in the second and third NWTS studies who developed congestive heart failure was 1.7% at 15 years after diagnosis; the percentage increased to 5.4% among those whose treatment included whole lung irradiation.[43] Late onset congestive heart failure may occasionally be precipitated by physiological stress, such as pregnancy.

Long-term survivors of Wilms tumor have been shown in several studies to have compensatory hypertrophy of the remaining kidney.[44-46] While post-nephrectomy hypertrophy is not influenced by the administration of adjuvant chemotherapy, it is decreased in patients who received whole-abdomen irradiation. The frequency of functional impairment is dose-related. Also, renal function may be impaired following irradiation of the extrarenal segment of the renal artery due to arterial stenosis, direct renal parenchymal irradiation and/or the administration of nephrotoxic chemotherapeutic agents. Although hypertension does not occur more frequently in long-term survivors of Wilms tumor than in the general population, Wilms tumor patients found to be hypertensive should be thoroughly evaluated for treatable causes of hypertension.

Both ovarian function and testicular function may fail following whole abdominal irradiation.[47,48] Testicular function may also be damaged by chemotherapy. Several groups have reported that pregnancy outcome is adversely affected by abdominal irradiation for Wilms tumor, i.e. lower birthweights and more perinatal deaths have been noted in these patients.[49] However, no increase in the frequency of congenital anomalies has been noted.

Second malignancies (SMNs), including leukemias and carcinomas, have been reported in children previously treated for Wilms tumor.[50,51] The frequency of SMNs in a cohort of successfully treated patients with Wilms tumor is approximately 5-10% 20 years after diagnosis.[50] The oncogenic effect of chemotherapy and irradiation may affect especially patients who are at risk of malignant transformation due to an inherited genetic defect.

Today, a major objective of those caring for children with Wilms tumor has become the modulation of treatment according to perceived risks of relapse, with the goal to reduce predictable side effects associated with anticancer treatment. Therefore, careful lifetime follow-up of these patients is indicated.

ASSOCIATED CONGENITAL ANOMALIES

The association of several genetically determined congenital anomalies with Wilms tumor has been of great use in identifying hereditary forms of Wilms tumor and in determining the chromosomal locations of genes involved in its etiology (see chapter 3).

GENITOURINARY ANOMALIES

With an incidence of 4-8%,[52] genitourinary anomalies are the most frequently reported congenital defects in patients with Wilms tumor. Yet, at the same time, they are the most overlooked and poorly delineated of the clinical phenotypes that should prompt monitoring for Wilms tumor. Genitourinary malformations associated with Wilms tumor include defects of the kidney (horseshoe kidney, fused kidney, renal dysplasia, renal aplasia, bilateral cystic kidney disease, chronic glomerulonephritis, nephrotic syndrome), hypospadias, cryptorchidism and duplication of the renal collecting system. Disorders like cryptorchidism and hypospadias, whose rate in Wilms tumor is only increased two-fold over the background rates, are so common in the pediatric population that "clinicians tend to focus on treating the anatomic problem rather than on searching for a syndrome diagnosis."[2] However, at present it is not clear which genitourinary malformations should trigger careful screening for Wilms tumor or extensive molecular genetic evaluation. The recent implication of the *WT1* gene in normal genitourinary development[53-56] (see also chapters 5 and 7) which could explain the association between Wilms tumor and genitourinary anomalies, clearly offers an invitation to address this issue.

ANIRIDIA AND WAGR SYNDROME

Aniridia (Fig. 1.3), the congenital absence of a part or all of the iris, shows a strong association with Wilms tumor. While the frequency of aniridia in the general population is 1:50,000 to 1:100,000, several studies have demonstrated that aniridia occurs in 1% of patients with Wilms tumor.[11,52] The association of aniridia and Wilms tumor has not only helped clinicians to identify a group of children at risk for the development of Wilms tumor, but has proved instrumental in locating the Wilms tumor suppressor gene *WT1*. From the clinical point, it has been suggested that patients with sporadic aniridia should be monitored for Wilms tumor, even if chromosome studies and phenotype are otherwise normal.[2] However, the majority of aniridia patients are those with the autosomal dominant form of this eye disease and do not have an increased risk for Wilms tumor.

HEMIHYPERTROPHY

Hemihypertrophy (Fig. 1.4) can be demonstrated in 2-3% of patients with Wilms tumor,[11,52] a significant increase over the background rate of 0.03/1,000. This increased frequency in Wilms tumor led to the suggestion of a congenital growth factor excess playing a role in the pathophysiology of both diseases, i.e. a "hyperplastic-neoplastic diathesis."[57] Thus far there is no direct evidence in support of this hypothesis. However, a recent epidemiologic study that demonstrated increased birth weights of children with Wilms tumor does suggest that growth factors present

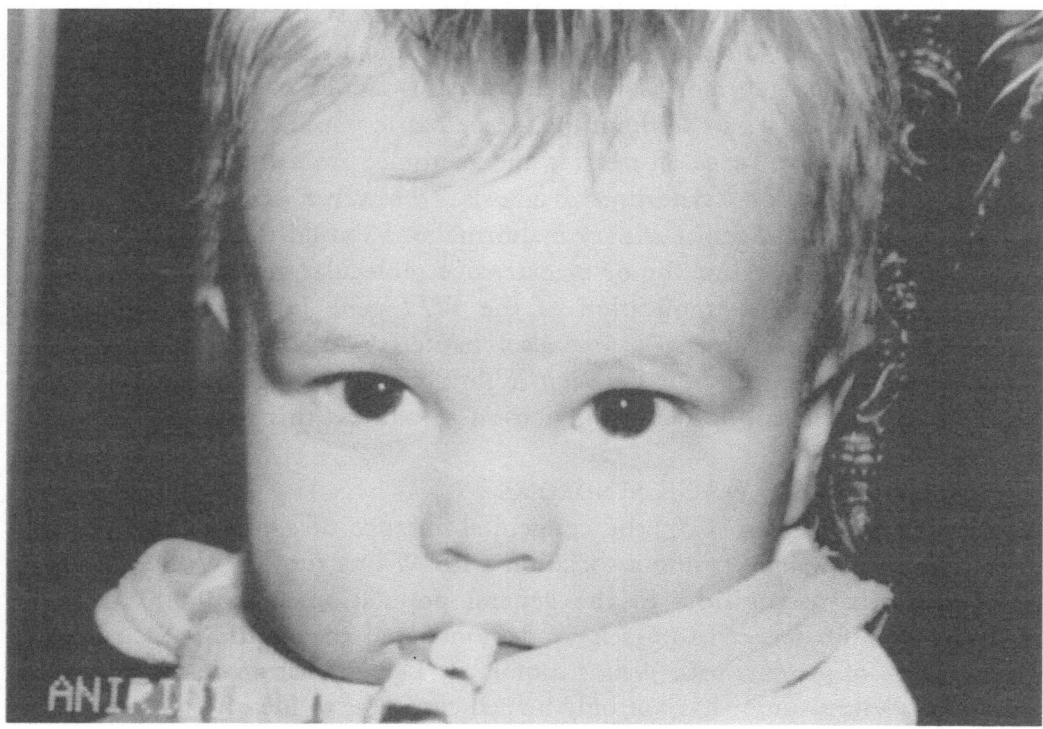

Fig. 1.3. Bilateral aniridia. As demonstrated in this figure, with this developmental anomaly, there is almost complete absence of the iris. The defect is usually accompanied by photophobia, nystagmus and defective vision. The condition may be familial or sporadic. This patient harbors a germline PAX6 mutation. Courtesy Dr. Carey Johnson, Department of Medical Genetics, University of Calgary and Alberta Children's Hospital, Calgary, Alberta.

prenatally may affect the development of Wilms tumor.[58] There is also growing epidemiologic and pathologic evidence that Wilms tumors associated with hemihypertrophy (and Beckwith-Wiedemann syndrome), differ from the tumors associated with the WAGR syndrome or the Denys-Drash syndrome.

BECKWITH-WIEDEMANN SYNDROME (BWS)

Closely related to hemihypertrophy is the Beckwith-Wiedemann syndrome (BWS) (Fig. 1.5), an overgrowth syndrome characterized by visceromegaly, macroglossia and hyperinsulinemic hypoglycemia. The heritability of BWS has been established, but the pattern of inheritance remains to be clarified. Possibilities include

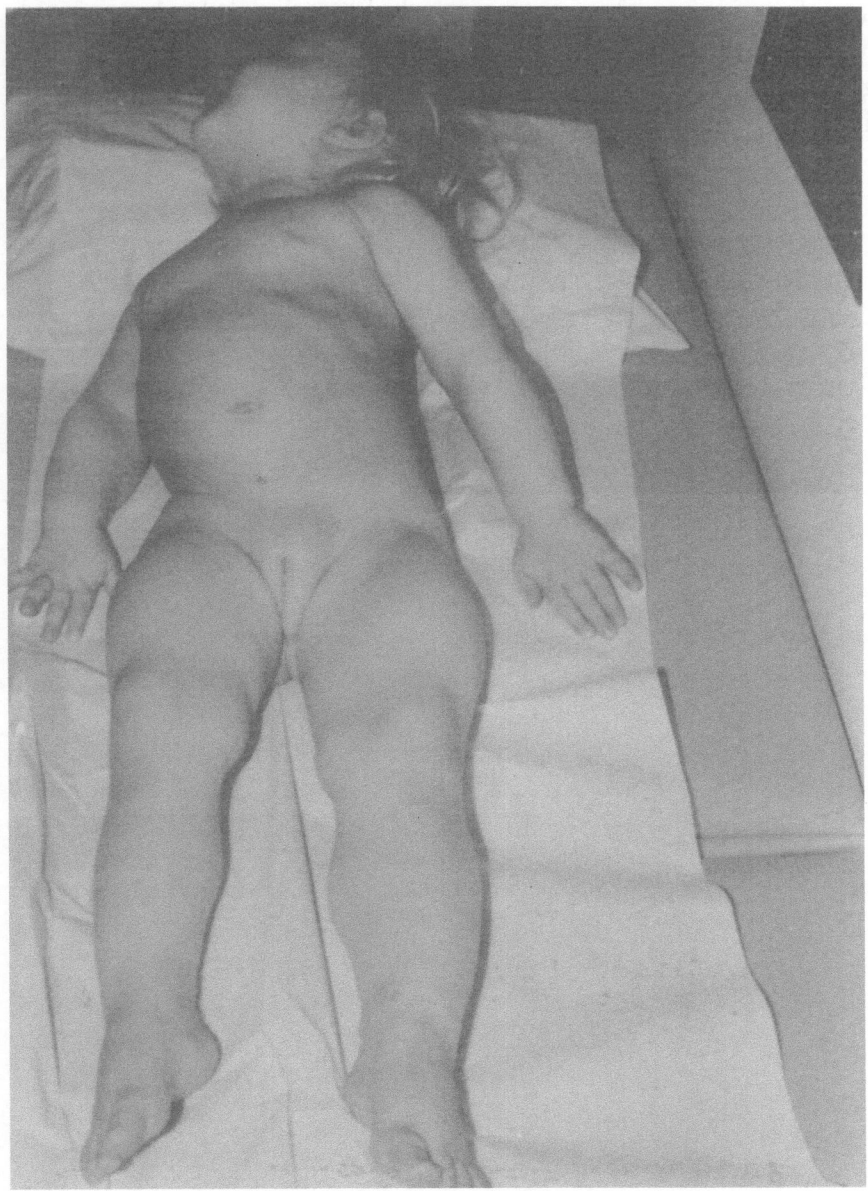

Fig. 1.4. Hemihypertrophy. Females are affected more often than males. The difference of the two sides (left > right) is usually greatest in the extremities, the genitalia and the trunk. Hemihypertrophy is a variable feature of Beckwith-Wiedemann syndrome. Courtesy Dr. Carey Johnson, Department of Medical Genetics, University of Calgary and Alberta Children's Hospital, Calgary, Alberta.

autosomal dominant inheritance with variable expression and reduced penetrance[59] and autosomal dominant inheritance with premutation such that only "carrier" females can produce the first generation of affected offspring.[60] Several other modes of inheritance have also been suggested and this disorder may prove to be

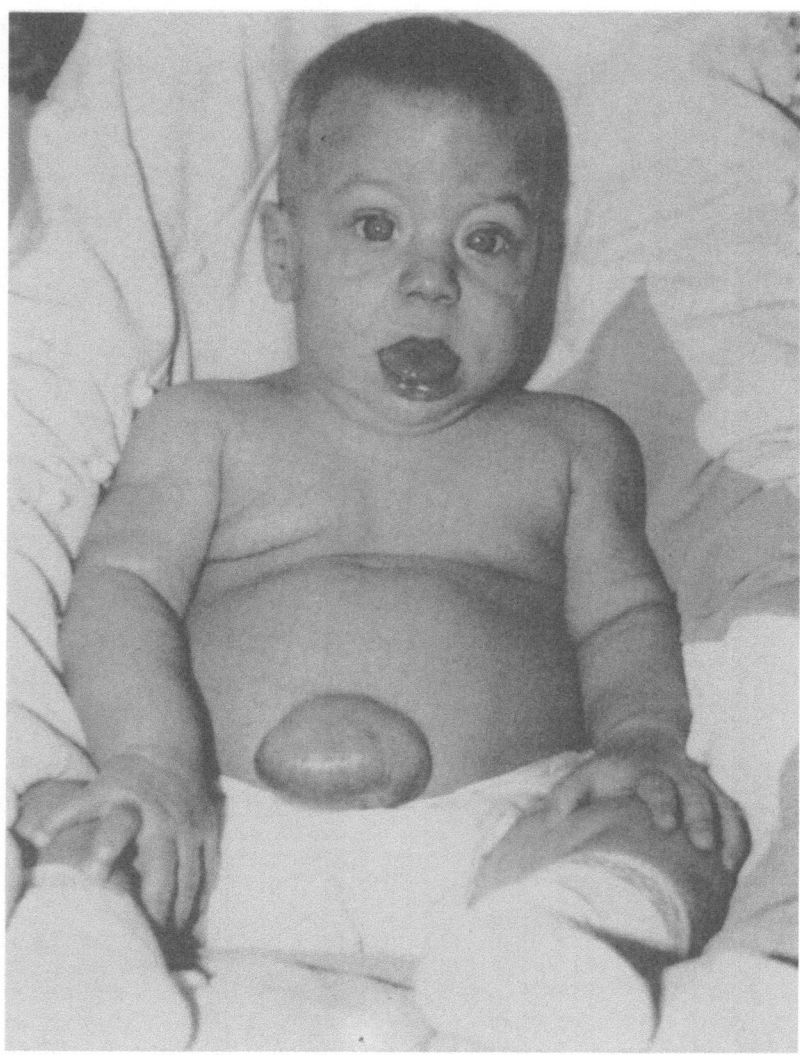

Fig. 1.5. Beckwith-Wiedemann syndrome. Beckwith-Wiedemann syndrome is characterized by numerous growth abnormalities, including enlarged tongue (macroglossia), gigantism, exomphalos and organomegaly. Courtesy Dr. Carey Johnson, Department of Medical Genetics, University of Calgary and Alberta Children's Hospital, Calgary, Alberta.

etiologically heterogeneous.[2] A possible explanation for the association of Wilms tumor with BWS was provided by the demonstrated linkage between the gene for familial BWS and chromosome 11p15,[61] a region frequently affected by loss of heterozygosity in sporadic Wilms tumor[62] (see chapter 8).

DENYS-DRASH SYNDROME (DDS)

Infrequently, Wilms tumor is associated with pseudohermaphroditism and nephropathy, a combination referred to as Denys-Drash syndrome (DDS).[63] Since some children have only two of the three characteristics of DDS, it has been suggested that the etiology of Wilms tumor, pseudohermaphroditism and nephropathy may be closely linked. Only children with all three disease features are considered to have DDS. The histologic features of the nephropathy are characteristic (Fig. 1.6) and consist of varying degrees of focal or diffuse mesangial sclerosis, usually occurring before the age of two years.[64] Because of the clinical overlap between this syndrome and the WAGR syndrome, it was suggested that the DDS too could arise as a consequence of a deletion of one or more genes localized at chromosome 11p13. This suggestion now has been confirmed. Germline mutations in the *WT1* gene have been shown to be responsible for DDS (see chapter 7).

OTHER ANOMALIES

Neurofibromatosis, an autosomal dominant inherited disease, has also been associated with Wilms tumor. Patients with Wilms tumor seem to have a marked increased incidence of neurofibromatosis,[65] although the limited number of patients studied indicates the need to interpret the available data with some caution. Additional anomalies associated with Wilms tumor include anomalies of the central nervous system, the musculoskeletal system, the cardiopulmonary system, the eye (excluding aniridia), and of hair, skin and nails.[52] Wilms tumor has also been associated with a rare form of dwarfism,[66] a syndrome that has an autosomal recessive inheritance and thus far has only been identified in Scandinavia.[67]

REFERENCES

1. Green DM, D'Angio GJ, Beckwith JB, Breslow N, Finklestein J, Kelalis P, Thomas P: Wilms' tumor (Nephroblastoma, renal embryoma). In: Pizzo PA and Poplack DG (eds): Principles and

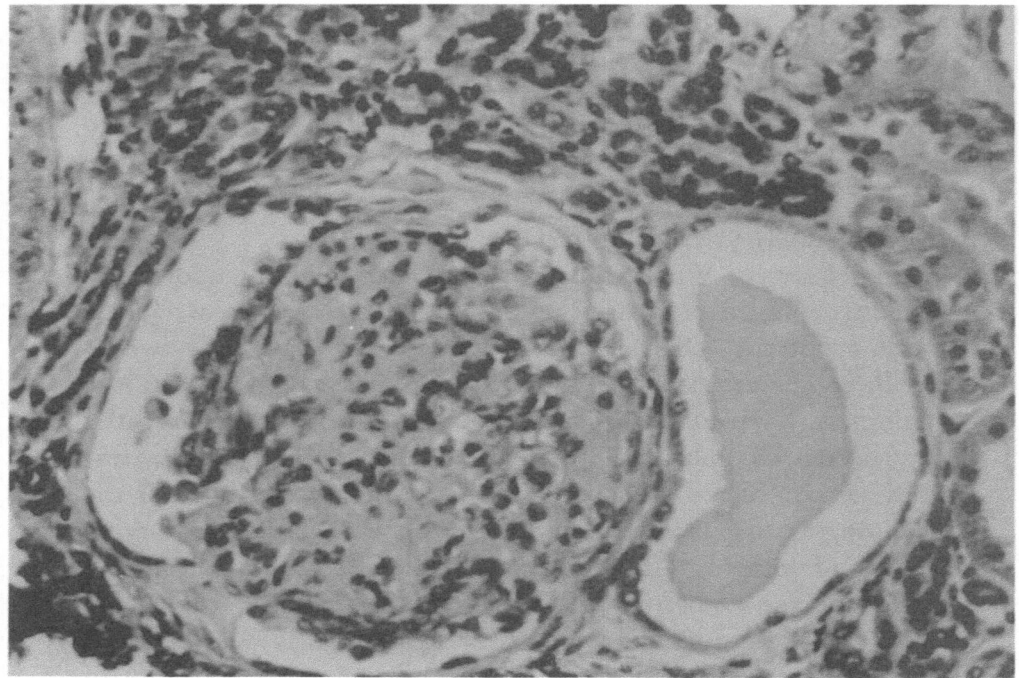

Fig. 1.6. Nephropathy in Denys-Drash syndrome. Photomicrographs of a normal glomerulus (A) and a glomerulus of a patient with Denys-Drash syndrome (B). The affected glomerulus shows mesangial cellular proliferation. Courtesy Dr. J. Carlos Manivel, Department of Laboratory Medicine and Pathology, University of Minnesota Hospitals and Clinics, Minneapolis, Minnesota. Reprinted with permission from M.J. Coppes, V. Huff and J. Pelletier, Denys-Drash syndrome: relating a clinical disorder to genetic alterations in the tumor suppressor gene WT1, J Pediatrics 1993; 123:673-678, copyright © Mosby-Year Book, Inc.

Practice of Pediatric Oncology. Philadelphia: J.B. Lippincott Company, 1993:713-737.

2. Clericuzio CL: Clinical phenotypes and Wilms tumor. Med and Pediatr Oncol, 1993; 21:182-187.

3. Clericuzio CL, D'Angio GJ, Duncan M, Green DM, Knudson Jr AG: Summary and recommendations of the workshop held at the first international conference on molecular and clinical genetics of childhood renal tumors, Albuquerque, New Mexico, May 14-16, 1992. Med Pediatr Oncol 1993; 21:233-236.

4. Breslow N, Olshan A, Beckwith JB, Green DM: Epidemiology of Wilms tumor. Med Pediatr Oncol 1993; 21:172-181.

5. Stiller CA, Parkin DM: International variations in the incidence of childhood renal tumours. Br J Cancer 1990; 62:1026-30.

6. Coppes MJ: Wilms tumor: A compilation of clinical and molecular characteristics. PhD thesis Amsterdam, 1992.

7. Kramer S, Meadows AT, Jarrett P: Racial variation in incidence of Wilms' tumor: relationship to congenital anomalies. Med Pediatr Oncol 1984; 12:401-405.

8. Breslow NE, Langholz B: Childhood cancer incidence: Geographical and temporal variations. Int J Cancer 1983; 32:703-716.

9. Arrigo S, Beckwith JB, Sharples K, D'Angio G, Haase G: Better survival after combined modality care for adults with Wilms' tumor. A report from the National Wilms' Tumor Study. Cancer 1990; 66:827-830.

10. Breslow N, Beckwith JB, Ciol M, Sharples K: Age distribution of Wilms' tumor: Report from the National Wilms' Tumor Study. Cancer Res 1988; 48:1653-1657.

11. Pastore G, Carli M, Lemerle J, Tournade MF, Voûte PA, Rey A, Burgers JMV, Zucker JM, Bürger D, De Kraker J, Delemarre JFM: Epidemiological features of Wilms' tumor: Results of studies by the International Society of Paediatric Oncology (SIOP). Med Pediatr Oncol 1988; 16:7-11.

12. Coppes MJ, De Kraker J, Van Dijken PJ, Perry HJ, Delemarre JF, Tournade MF, Lemerle J, Voûte PA: Bilateral Wilms' tumor: Long-term survival and some epidemiological features. J Clin Oncol 1989; 7:310-315.

13. Shearer P, Parham DM, Fontanesi J, Kumar M, Lobe TE, Fairclough D, Douglass EC, Wilimas J: Bilateral Wilms tumor. Cancer 1993; 72:1422-1426.

14. Knudson AG, Strong LC: Mutation and cancer: A model for Wilms' tumor of kidney. J Natl Cancer Inst 1972; 48:313-324.

15. Bunin GR, Kramer S, Marrero O, Meadows AT: Gestational risk factors for Wilms' tumor: Results of a case-control study. Cancer Res 1987; 47:2972-2977.

16. Bunin GR, Nass CC, Kramer S, Meadows AT: Parental occupation and Wilms' tumor: Results of a case-control study. Cancer Res 1989; 49:725-729.

17. Coppes MJ: Serum biological markers and paraneoplastic syndromes in Wilms tumor. Med Pediatr Oncol 1993; 21:213-221.

18. Green DM: Diagnosis and management of malignant solid tumors in infants and children. Boston: Martinus Nijhoff Publishing, 1985.

19. Coppes MJ, Zandvoort SW, Sparling CR, Poon AO, Weitzman S, Blanchette VS: Acquired von Willebrand disease in Wilms' tumor patients. J Clin Oncol 1992; 10:422-427.

20. Kenny GM, Mirand EA, Staubitz WJ, Allen JE, Trudel PJ, Murphy GP: Erythropoietin levels in Wilms tumor patients. J Urol 1970;; 104:758-761.

21. Murphy GP, Allen JE, Staubitz WJ, Sinks LF, Mirand EA: Erythropoietin levels in patients with Wilms tumor. Follow-up evaluation. NY State J Med 1972; 72:487-489.

22. Tsuchida Y, Mochida Y, Kamii Y, Honna T, Saeki M, Hata J,

Yokoyama T, Sasaki F, Nishiura M, Takeda K, et al: Determination of plasma total renin level by RIA with a monoclonal antibody: value as a marker for nephroblastoma. J Pediatr Surg 1990; 25:1092-1094.

23. Tsuchida Y, Yokomori K, Nishiuria M, Shimizu K: Total renin as a marker for pediatric tumours. Med Pediatr Oncol 1993; 21:603.

24. Kumar S, West DC, Ponting JM, Gattamaneni HR: Sera of children with renal tumours contain low-molecular-mass hyaluronic acid. Int J Cancer 1989; 44:445-448.

25. Longaker MT, Adzick NS, Sadigh D, Hendin B, Stair SE, Duncan BW, Harrison MR, Spendlove R, Stern R: Hyaluronic acid-stimulating activity in the pathophysiology of Wilms' tumors. J Natl Cancer Inst 1990; 82:135-139.

26. Stern M, Longaker MT, Adzick NS, Harrison MR, Stern R: Hyaluronidase levels in urine from Wilms' tumor patients. J Natl Cancer Inst 1991; 83:1569-1574.

27. D'Angio GJ, Rosenberg H, Sharples K, Kelalis P, Breslow N, Green DM: Position paper: Imaging methods for primary renal tumors of childhood: Costs versus benefits. Med Pediatr Oncol 1993; 21:205-212.

28. Thomas PR, Shochat SJ, Norkool P, Beckwith JB, Breslow NE, D'Angio GJ: Prognostic implications of hepatic adhesion, invasion, and metastases at diagnosis of Wilms' tumor. The National Wilms' Tumor Study Group. Cancer 1991; 68:2486-2488.

29. Ritchey ML, Othersen HJ, De Lorimier A, Kramer SA, Benson C, Kelalis PP: Renal vein involvement with nephroblastoma: A report of the National Wilms' Tumor Study-3. Eur Urol 1990; 17: 139-144.

30. Beahrs OH, Henson DE, Hutter RVP, Myers MH: Manual for staging of cancer. Philadelphia: JB Lippincott Company, 1988.

31. Tournade MF, Com-Nougué C, Voûte PA, Lemerle J, De Kraker J, Delemarre JFM, Burgers M, Habrand JL, Moorman CGM, Bürger D, Rey A, Zucker JM, Carli M, Jereb B, Bey P, Gauthier F, Sandstedt B: Results of the sixth International Society of Pediatric Oncology Wilms' tumor trial and study: A risk-adapted therapeutic approach in Wilms' tumor. J Clin Oncol 1993; 11: 1014-1023.

32. Ladd WE, White RR: Embryoma of the kidney (Wilms' tumor). JAMA 1941; 117:1858-1862.

33. Ehrlich RM: Complications of Wilms'tumor surgery. Urol Clin North Amer 1983; 10:399-406.

34. D'Angio GJ, Evans AE, Breslow N, Beckwith B, Bishop H, Faigl P, Goodwin W, Leape LL, Sinks LF, Sutow W, Tefft M, Wolff J: The treatment of Wilms' tumor. Results from the National Wilms' Tumor Study. Cancer 1976; 38:633-646.

35. Lemerle J, Voûte PA, Tournade MF, Rodary C, Delemarre JFM, Sarrazin D, Burgers JMV, Sandstedt B, Middenberger H, Carli M,

Jereb B, C.G.M. M-V: Effectiveness of preoperative chemotherapy in Wilms' tumor: Results of an International Society of Paediatric Oncology (SIOP) clinical trial. J Clin Oncol 1983; 10:604-609.

36. D'Angio GJ, Breslow N, Beckwith JB, Evans A, Baum H, DeLorimier A, Fernbach D, Hrabovsky E, Jones B, Kelalis P, Othersen B, Tefft M, Thomas PRM: Treatment of Wilms' tumor. Results of the Third National Wilms' Tumor Study. Cancer 1989; 64:349-360.

37. Thomas PR, Tefft M, Compaan PJ, Norkool P, Breslow NE, D'Angio GJ: Results of two radiation therapy randomizations in the third National Wilms' Tumor Study. Cancer 1991; 68:1703-7.

38. D'Angio GJ, Farber S, Maddock CL: Potentiation of x-ray effects of actinomycin D. Radiology 1959; 73:175-177.

39. Sutow W, Thurman WG, Windmiller J: Vincristine (leucocristine) sulfate in the treatment of children with metastatic Wilms' tumor. Pediatrics 1963; 32:880-887.

40. Bellani FF, Gasparini M, Boanadonna G: Adriamycin in Wilm's tumor previously treated with chemotherapy. Eur J Cancer Clin Oncol 1975; 11:593-595.

41. Evans AE, Norkool P, Evans I, Breslow N, D'Angio GJ: Late effects of treatment for Wilms' tumor. A report from the National Wilms' Tumor Study Group. Cancer 1991; 67:331-336.

42. Von Hoff DD, Layard MW, Basa P, Davis Jr HL, Von Hoff AL, Rozencwig M, Muggio FM: Risk factors for doxorubicin-induced congestive heart failure. Ann Int Med 1979; 91:710-717.

43. Green DM, Breslow NE, Moksness J D, D'Angio, GJ: Congestive heart failure following initial therapy for Wilms tumor. A report from the National Wilms tumor study. Pediatr Res 1994; 35:161A.

44. Luttenegger TJ, Gooding CA, Fickenscher LG: Compensatory renal hypertrophy after treatment for Wilms' tumor. Am J Roentgenol 1975; 125:348-351.

45. Walker RD, Reid CF, Richard GA, Talbert JL, Rogers BM: Compensatory renal growth and function in post-nephrectomized patients with Wilms' tumor. Urology 1982; 19:127-130.

46. Wikstad I, Celsi G, Larsson L, Herin P, Aperia A: Kidney function in adults born with unilateral agenesis or nephrectomized in childhood. Pediatr Nephrol 1988; 2:177-182.

47. Shalet SM, Beardwell CG, Morris-Jones PH, Pearson D, Orrell DH: Ovarian function following abdominal irradiation in childhood. Br J Cancer 1976; 33:655-658.

48. Shalet SM, Beardwell CG, Jacobs HS, Pearson D: Testicular function following irradiation of the human prepubertal testis. Clin Endocrinol 1978; 9:483-490.

49. Li FP, Gimbrere K, Gelber RD, Sallan SE, Flamant F, Green DM, Heyn RM, Meadows AT: Outcome of pregnancy in survivors of Wilms' tumor. JAMA 1987; 257:216-219.

50. Li FP, Yan JC, Sallan S, Cassady JR, Danahy J, Fine W, Gelber RD, Green DM: Second neoplasms after Wilms' tumor in childhood. J Nat Cancer Inst 1983; 71:1205-1209.
51. Breslow NE, Norkool PA, Olshan A, Evans A, D'Angio GJ: Second malignant neoplasms in survivors of Wilms' tumor: A report from the National Wilms' Tumor Study. J Natl Cancer Inst 1988; 80:592-595.
52. Breslow NE, Beckwith JB: Epidemiological features of Wilms' tumor: Results of the National Wilms' Tumor Study. J Natl Cancer Inst 1982; 68:429-436.
53. Van Heyningen V, Bickmore WA, Seawright A, Fletcher JM, Maule J, Fekete G, Gessler M, Bruns GA, Huerre-Jeanpierre C, Junien C, Williams BRG, Hastie ND: Role for the Wilms tumor gene in genital development? Proc Natl Acad Sci USA 1990; 87:5383-5386.
54. Pelletier J, Bruening W, Li FP, Haber DA, Glaser T, Housman DE: *WT1* mutations contribute to abnormal genital system development and hereditary Wilms' tumour. Nature 1991; 353:431-434.
55. Pelletier J, Schalling M, Buckler AJ, Rogers A, Haber DA, Housman D: Expression of the Wilms' tumor gene *WT1* in the murine urogenital system. Genes Dev 1991; 5:1345-1356.
56. Kreidberg JA, Sarlola H, Loring JM, Maeda M, Pelletier J, Housman D, Jaenish R: WT-1 is required for early kidney development. Cell 1993; 74:679-691.
57. Miller RW, Fraumeni JF, Manning MD: Association of Wilms's tumor with aniridia, hemihypertrophy and other congenital abnormalities. N Engl J Med 1964; 270:922-927.
58. Leisenring WM, Breslow NE, Evans IE, Beckwith JB, Coppes MJ, Grundy P: Increased birth weights of National Wilms Tumor Study patients suggest a growth factor excess. Cancer Res 1994; 54:4680-4683.
59. Niikawa N, Ishikiriyama S, Takahashi S, Inagawa A, Tonoki H, Ohta Y, Hase N, Kamei T, Kajii T: The Wiedemann-Beckwith syndrome; Pedigree studies on five families with evidence for autosomal dominant inheritance with variable expressivity. Am J Med Genet 1986; 24:41-55.
60. Aleck KA, Hadro TA: Dominant inheritance of Wiedemann-Beckwith syndrome: Further evidence for transmission of "unstable permutation" through carrier women. Am J Med Genet 1989; 33:155-160.
61. Koufos A, Grundy P, Morgan K, Aleck KA, Hadro T, Lampkin BC, Kalbakji A, Cavenee WK: Familial Wiedemann-Beckwith syndrome and a second Wilms tumor locus both map to 11p15.5. Am J Hum Genet 1989; 44:711-719.
62. Coppes MJ, Bonetta L, Huang A, Hoban P, Chilton-MacNeill S, Campbell CE, Weksberg R, Yeger H, Reeve AE, Williams BRG: Loss of heterozygosity mapping in Wilms tumor indicates the in-

volvement of three distinct regions and a limited role for non-disjunction or mitotic recombination. Genes Chrom Cancer 1992; 5:326-334.

63. Jadresic L, Leake J, Gordon I, Dillon MJ, Grant DB, Pritchard J, Risdon RA, Barratt TM: Clinicopathologic review of twelve children with nephropathy, Wilms tumor, and genital abnormalities (Drash syndrome). J Pediat 1990; 117:717-725.

64. Habib R, Loirat C, Gubler MC, Niaudet P, Bensman A, Levy M, Broyer M: The nephropathy associated with male pseudohermaphroditism and Wilms' tumor (Drash syndrome): A distinctive glomerular lesion - report of 10 cases. Clin Nephrol 1985; 24:269-278.

65. Stay EJ, Vawter G: The relation between nephroblastoma and neurofibromatosis (Von Recklinghausen's disease). Cancer 1977; 39:2550-2555.

66. Simila S, Timonen M, Heikinnen E: A case of Mulibrey nanism with associated Wilms' tumor. Clin Genet 1980; 17:29-30.

67. Perheentupa J, Autio S, Leisti S, Raitta C, Tuuteri L: Mulibrey nanism, an autosomal recessive syndrome with pericardial constriction. Lancet 1973; ii:351-355.

CHAPTER 2

HISTOPATHOLOGY

INTRODUCTION

Since the first well-documented morphological descriptions of nephroblastoma,[1,2] which preceded Max Wilms' landmark monograph "Die Mischgeschwülste der Niere"[3] by two decades, information on the morphology of Wilms tumors has accumulated rapidly. Histopathologic studies conducted under the auspices of both the North American National Wilms Tumor Study (NWTS) and the European International Society of Paediatric Oncology (SIOP) have resulted in an extensive body of literature concerning the histomorphology of this childhood neoplasm. Traditionally viewed as a triphasic embryonal renal tumor, it is now clear that some Wilms tumors may be biphasic or even monomorphic, causing some differential diagnostic challenges. This chapter intends to provide a basic understanding of some of the histopathologic features of childhood renal tumors, including Wilms tumor.

WILMS TUMOR

GROSS APPEARANCE

Usually Wilms tumor presents as a massive multilobulated solitary solid tumor (Fig. 2.1), originating from any part of either kidney. Most Wilms tumors are unicentric lesions that replace normal renal parenchyma and distort the renal outline. Compression and scarring of the surrounding tissues produces a gross appearance of encapsulation (pseudocapsule), a feature that may help to distinguish Wilms tumor from other renal tumors such as mesoblastic nephroma, clear cell sarcoma, rhabdoid tumor and renal lymphoma.[4] The parenchyma of most Wilms tumors is pale

Wilms Tumor: Clinical and Molecular Characterization, by Max J. Coppes, Christine E. Campbell, and Bryan R.G. Williams. © 1995 R.G. Landes Company.

gray or tan colored on section, but this may be altered by second-ary changes such as necrosis, hemorrhage, cystic formation or the accumulation of mucinous matrix. Calcification is not often present, although in approximately 10% of the cases it is of sufficient mag-nitude to be detected on plain films.[5] Multilobulation is an im-portant gross characteristic (Fig. 2.1), which needs to be distin-guished from multicentricity, a distinction that is not likely settled by macroscopic inspection of the surgical specimen, but requires careful microscopic evaluation.

MICROSCOPIC APPEARANCE

"Classic" Wilms tumor is composed of persistent blastema, dysplastic tubules, and supporting mesenchyme or stroma (Fig. 2.2). It is characterized by islands of compact undifferentiated blastema and the presence of variable epithelial differentiation in the form of

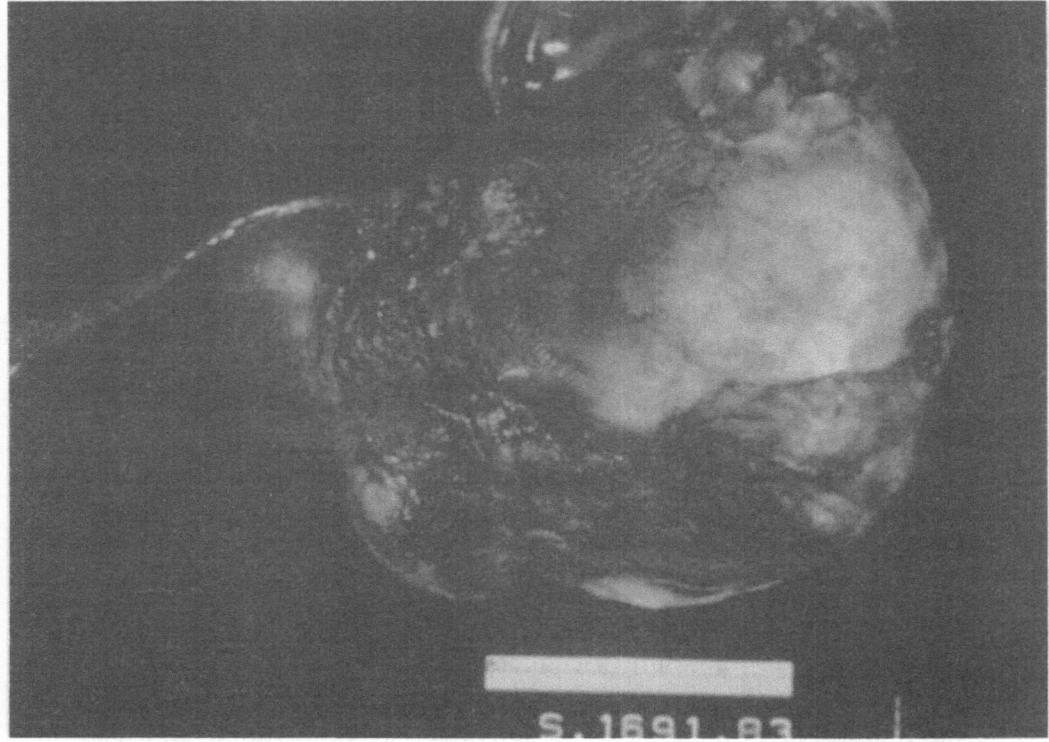

Fig. 2.1. Macroscopic appearance of Wilms tumor. While multilobulation is characteristic for Wilms tumor, macroscopically it cannot be distinguished from multicentricity. Microscopic analysis however enables the distinction to be made.

embryonic tubules, rosettes and glomeruloid structures separated by a significant stromal component. The proportion of each of these components vary from infrequent to abundant within and among individual tumors. Focal areas of atypical mesenchymal derived components, such as smooth and striated muscle, adipose tissue and, more rarely, cartilage or bone may also be observed[6] and have been attributed to aberrant differentiation of mesodermal metanephrogenic blastema. The coexistence of blastemal, epithelial and stromal cells has led to the term "triphasic" to characterize the histologic composition of "classic" Wilms tumor. Some Wilms tumors however, are not triphasic but present only biphasic or even monomorphous patterns.[6]

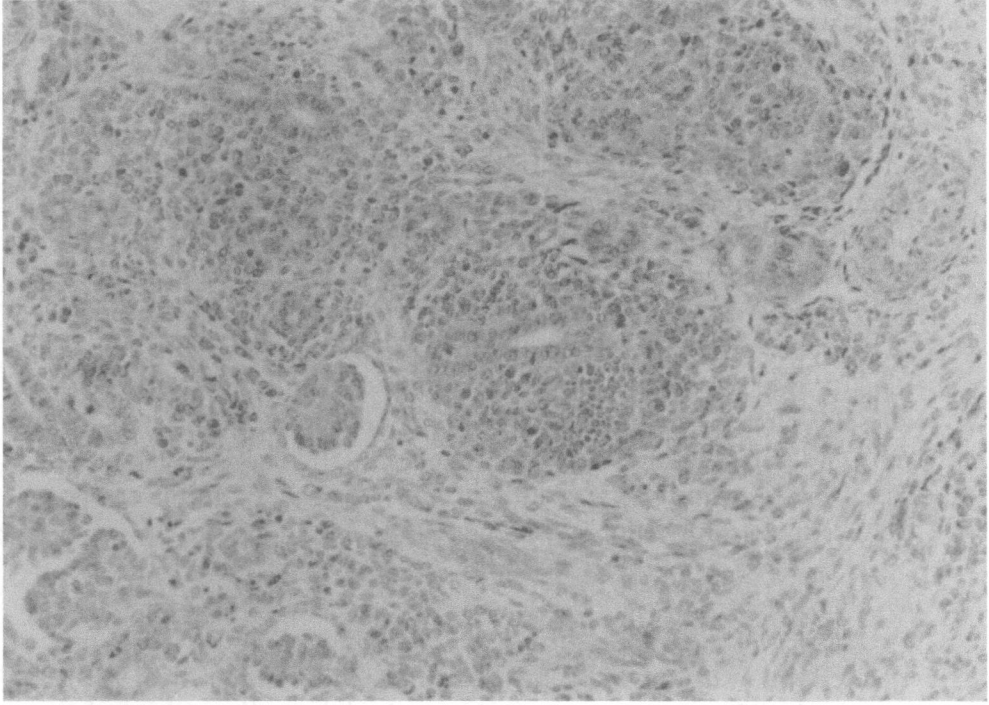

Fig. 2.2. Wilms tumor, favorable histology. This medium-magnification view shows the three cell categories usually present in Wilms tumor: (1) stromal cells are the loosely packed spindled cells, best seen in the upper left corner; (2) blastemal cells are the more compact polygonal cells such as those surrounding a tubule near the center; (3) epithelial cells are seen best in the center and toward the right side of the field where they form tubular or glomeruloid structures. Note the small size and regular shape of the nuclei, indicating the absence of anaplasia. Courtesy of Dr. J. Bruce Beckwith, Department of Pathology, Loma Linda University, California. Reprinted with permission from M.J. Coppes, Wilms tumor: From cure to understanding, Critical Reviews in Oncology and Hematology 1995; 18:179-196. Copyright © Elsevier Scientific Publishers, Ireland Ltd.

Ultrastructural, immunohistochemical, and other special diagnostic studies are rarely used in the diagnosis of Wilms tumor since this childhood cancer infrequently presents difficulties in recognition. When only a very small biopsy specimen is available for diagnosis, or the lesion is extremely undifferentiated, such studies may be helpful. Ultrastructurally, Wilms tumor is characterized by numerous well-developed desmosomes, prominent cilia, and various amounts of amorphous electron-dense extracellular deposits usually clinging to the external surface of the tumor cells.[7] Immunohistochemical studies are primarily used to rule out other primitive childhood tumors.[8]

The structural diversity of Wilms tumor has allowed the study of certain histopathologic features to determine if any of these correlate with outcome. Epithelial differentiation has been the subject of some study. Although not as significant as the absence of "unfavorable characteristics," tubular differentiation has been recognized as a histologic feature correlating with young age of onset and favorable outcome.[9-11] However, examples of aggressive Wilms tumors featuring monomorphous tubular histology[10] have prevented the classification of this distinct morphologic entity as a truly favorable characteristic. Also, as more effective therapeutic regimens have increased overall survival, it has become difficult to discriminate between the more favorable variants; only the unfavorable ones remain as a distinctive subgroup.[12] Markers associated with unfavorable outcome include focal and diffuse nuclear atypia (anaplasia), and sarcomatous tumors ("rhabdoid" and "clear cell" type). The latter two tumor types are currently viewed as tumor categories distinct from Wilms tumor.

ANAPLASIA

Anaplasia, a major indicator of poor outcome,[13] was first recognized in Wilms tumor by Beckwith and Palmer in 1978.[14] Anaplastic Wilms tumors are characterized by cells with nuclear enlargement to three or more times the diameter of adjacent cells, hyperchromasia of enlarged nuclei and abnormal mitotic figures (Fig. 2.3). The overall incidence of anaplasia varies from 3.2% to 7.3%.[13,15,16] It is rarely seen in tumors of patients <2 years of age at diagnosis (incidence about 2%) but its presence increases to a relatively stable incidence of about 13% in those >5 years of age.[4] Initially its distribution by sex was reported to be

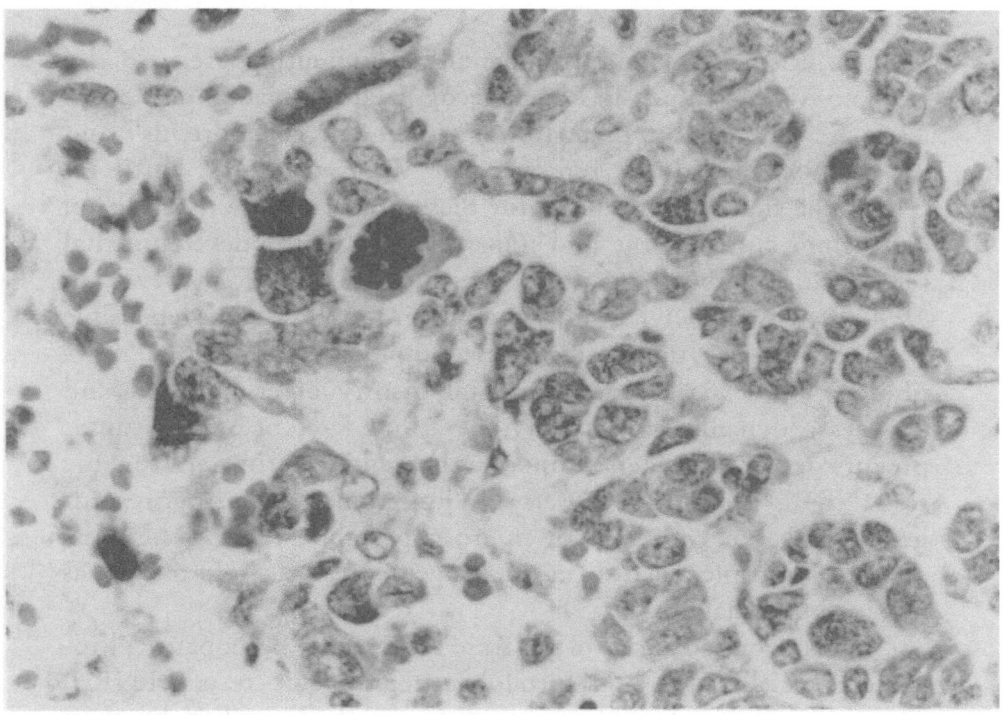

Fig. 2.3. Wilms tumor with anaplasia. This high-magnification photograph shows marked variation in size, shape and density of nuclei. Note especially the multipolar mitotic figure to the right of center, and the large, densely-stained nucleus to its right. These findings indicate the presence of extreme polyploidy in some nuclei. Courtesy of Dr. J. Bruce Beckwith, Department of Pathology, Loma Linda University, California. Reprinted with permission from M.J. Coppes, Wilms tumor: From cure to understanding, Critical Reviews in Oncology and Hematology 1995; 18:179-196. Copyright © Elsevier Scientific Publishers, Ireland Ltd.

equal but recent publications suggest a higher incidence in female patients.[16] Finally, its incidence is significantly higher in non Caucasian patients.[13]

If anaplasia is found in less than 10% of the microscopic fields at high dry magnification it is designated "focal," if it exceeds 10% it is labeled "diffuse." The presence of anaplasia carries a poor prognosis, especially for those patients with diffuse anaplastic advanced stage disease.[4] Recently, the classifications "diffuse" and "focal" have been redefined.[17] It remains to be determined how applicable this new classification is for general pathologists and whether it will enable a more accurate differentiation for those with a relatively good from those with an outright poor outcome.

NEPHROGENIC RESTS

The existence of lesions apparently representing precursor lesions to Wilms tumor has been recognized for several decades.[18] They are found in approximately 1% of infant postmortems[18] and 30 to 40% of kidneys removed for Wilms tumor.[19] Until recently, the nomenclature used for these precursor lesions has been confusing, cumbersome and non-reflective of the developmental relationships between the various lesional categories. However, in 1990, Beckwith, Kiviat and Bonadio proposed a comprehensible classification and terminology based on the principle that morphology reflects the developmental history of each lesion and conveys a dynamic concept of the various fates of Wilms tumor precursors.[20] Since their proposal, the generic term nephrogenic rest (NR) is used for all putative Wilms tumor precursors regardless of size, gross features or microscopic appearance. The presence of multiple or diffuse nephrogenic rests is referred to as nephro-blastomatosis.[20]

Two major categories of NRs are recognized: perilobar nephrogenic rests (PLNRs) and intralobar nephrogenic rests (ILNRs). These two types of nephrogenic rests are distinguished by their position within the renal lobe (Fig. 2.4), the organizational unit of the metanephros.[21,22] The renal lobe should not be confused with the renal lobule, the small cortical zone centered around a single medullary ray. Since there is a fundamental relationship between lobar topography and the chronology of renal development, relative position within the lobe is a direct reflection of the chronology of development. Because PLNRs are found in the lobar periphery only, while ILNRs are found anywhere within the lobe, as well as in the renal sinus and the wall of the pelvicaliceal system (Fig. 2.4), ILNRs generally reflect earlier developmental events than do PLNRs. Table 2.1 lists the principal morphological features of both rest types. Of particular note are the characteristically sharp margins of PLNRs and the irregular, interdigitating margins of most ILNRs. The fact that occasional rests defy categorization indicates some degree of overlap between the two categories, and suggests that ILNRs and PLNRs may represent opposite ends of a developmental continuum.[20] A more detailed subclassification of NRs can be found elsewhere.[20,23]

ILNRs and PLNRs are associated with different epidemiological features. For example, the age at diagnosis for children with

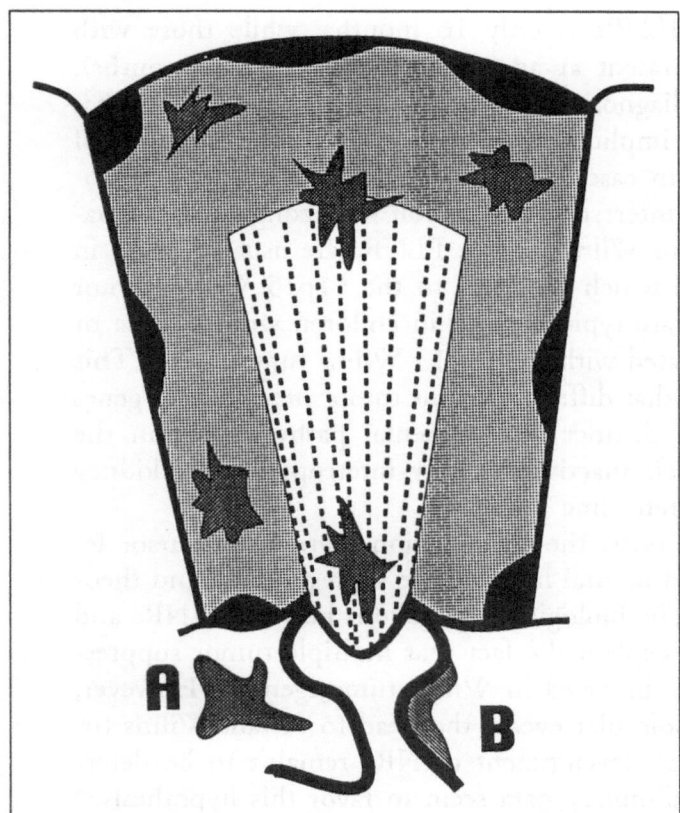

Fig. 2.4. Location of PLNRs and ILNRs within the renal lobe. Diagrammatic representation of a renal lobe, with an adjacent portion of renal sinus and pelviceal system, showing characteristic locations of PLNR (black) and ILNR (dark gray). A shows ILNR in a renal sinus. B shows ILNR in the wall of the calyx. Reprinted with permission from: J. Bruce Beckwith, Precursor lesions of Wilms tumor: Clinical and biological implications, Medical and Pediatric Oncology 1993; 21:158-168, © Wiley-Liss, a Division of John Wiley and Sons, Inc.

Table 2.1. Morphological features distinguishing ILNR from PLNR

	ILNR	PLNR
Position in lobe	Periphery	Random, including cortex, medulla, sinus, and caliceal wall
Number	Usually numerous	Usually sparse, often single,
Relations to adjacent nephrons	Demarcated, no nephrons inside rest	Interstitial, nephrons mingled with rest cells
Structure	Stroma sparse or sclerotic Blastemal or epithelial	Stroma usually prominent Blastema forms cuffs around tubules

From J. Bruce Beckwith, Precursor lesions of Wilms tumor: Clinical and biological implications, Medical and Pediatric Oncology 1993; 21:158-168. Copyright © Wiley-Liss, a Division of John Wiley and Sons, Inc.

Wilms tumor and ILNRs is only 16 months, while those with associated PLNRs present at an older median age (36 months). The median age at diagnosis of those without NRs is 41 months.[23] This difference has implications with respect to the duration of patient surveillance in cases of nephroblastomatosis. Also, categories of NR show an interesting association with congenital anomalies that predispose to Wilms tumor. PLNRs are usually found in children with BWS, which is linked to the 11p15 Wilms tumor locus, while ILNRs are typically seen in children with aniridia or other features associated with the 11p13 Wilms tumor locus. This observations suggest that different Wilms tumor predisposing genes may be involved in distinct developmental pathways within the kidney, and that their inactivation may interrupt normal kidney development at discrete time points.

The presence of NRs, the classification of these precursor lesions and their varied natural history have both practical and theoretical importance. The biological distinctions between ILNRs and PLNRs have helped explain the fact that multiple tumor suppressor genes seem to be involved in Wilms tumorigenesis. However, whether the same molecular events that lead to certain Wilms tumors also lead to the development of NRs remains to be determined, although preliminary data seem to favor this hypothesis.[24] Nevertheless, it remains possible that some precursor lesions are caused by genetic events different from the ones that are involved in the development of Wilms tumor in the same kidney. From the practical point of view on the finding of nephroblastomatosis should alert the physician to an increased likelihood of subsequent tumor development in the remaining renal parenchyma. As such the presence of nephroblastomatosis forms an indication for careful follow-up of the remaining renal tissue by appropriate imaging studies.

CONGENITAL MESOBLASTIC NEPHROMA

The recognition of congenital mesoblastic nephroma (CMN) as a distinct clinicopathologic entity with a more favorable outcome then Wilms tumor is ascribed to Bolande, Brough and Izant.[25] It occurs in approximately one of 500,000 infants and accounts for less than 3% of pediatric renal tumors. CMN usually is diagnosed in patients at birth or within the first three months of life,[26,27] as opposed to Wilms tumor that has a median age at diagnosis of

36 months. Characteristically, this tumor is firm, rubbery, dense and whitish. Unlike Wilms tumor, CMNs do not have a pseudo-capsule. The presence of cystic or pseudocystic areas due to necrosis[27] is not typical for CMN[5] but does not preclude its diagnosis.[28] Microscopically, these tumors are predominantly composed of bundles of spindle cells resembling fibroblasts or smooth muscle cells (Fig. 2.5). Ultrastructural studies have shown features consistent with the fibroblastic nature of the cells.[5]

The most important aspect of the recognition of these tumors as a separate entity is the usually excellent outcome of CMN with radical surgery only. During surgery, efforts must be made to secure the removal of a wide margin of uninvolved tissue.[28] The presence of increased cellularity, focal or diffuse, and high mitotic

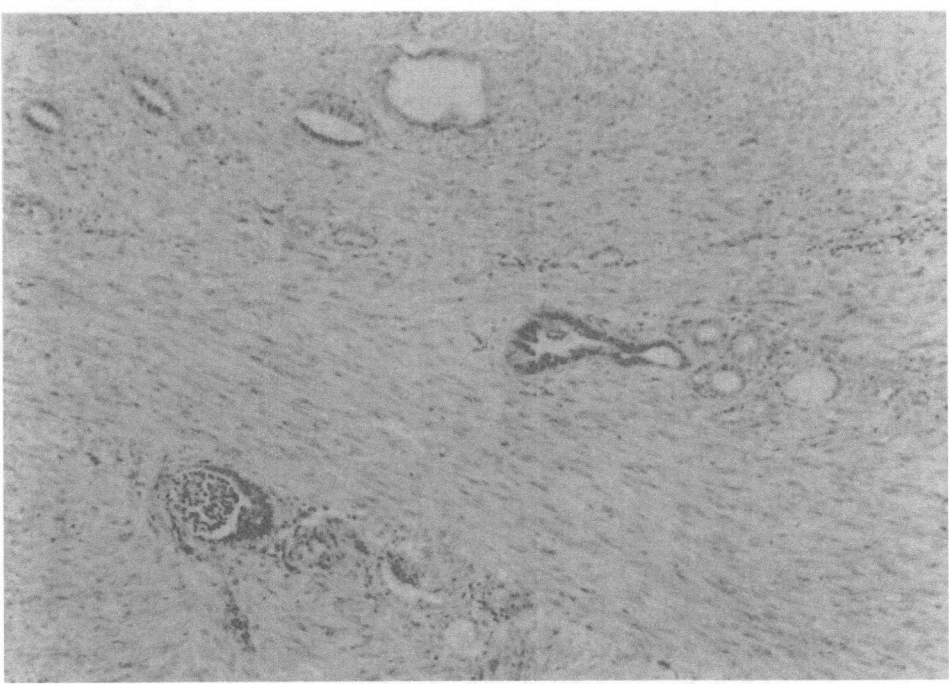

Fig. 2.5. Congenital mesoblastic nephroma (CMN). This medium-magnification view shows spindled tumor cells mingled with tubules and glomeruli. The latter are entrapped renal elements, and indicate the manner in which CMN interdigitates with adjacent normal structures. Entrapped renal elements are often misinterpreted as part of the neoplasm, and can lead to a mistaken diagnosis of Wilms tumor. Courtesy of Dr. J. Bruce Beckwith, Department of Pathology, Loma Linda University, California. Reprinted with permission from M.J. Coppes, Wilms tumor: From cure to understanding, Critical Reviews in Oncology and Hematology 1995; 18:179-196. Copyright © Elsevier Scientific Publishers, Ireland Ltd.

rate should however cause caution in infants over three months of age, as some patients with such lesions have had local recurrence and/or distal metastases.

Although both Wilms tumor and CMN arise from the developing kidney, it has been suggested that the key difference between the two may be the developmental time point at which the induction of neoplasia occurs.[29] Molecular analysis indicates that while Wilms tumor is frequently associated with LOH at chromosome bands 11p13 and/or 11p15,[30] CMNs, in a very limited number analyzed, are not.[31] The latter observation does not of course exclude the presence of subtle genetic alterations at *WT1* or *WT2* in CMNs.

CLEAR CELL SARCOMA OF THE KIDNEY

This variant was first described in 1970[32] and independently identified in 1978 by pathologists of the NWTS[14] and the UK Medical Research Council Nephroblastoma trial.[33] Clear cell sarcoma of the kidney (CCSK), or "bone metastasizing renal tumor of childhood,"[33] comprises about 4% of childhood renal tumors. Characteristically, the gross appearance of CCSK is that of a tan-colored tumor which may or may not present with some cysts. The light microscopic appearance (Fig. 2.6) is usually uniform and consists of abundant and evenly distributed fibrovascular stroma creating an alveolar or occasionally trabecular pattern.[34] This can easily be differentiated from the histologic features described in Wilms tumor, although a number of variant CCSK patterns can cause confusion. Bilateral involvement has thus far not been reported, nor has the presence of Wilms tumor associated congenital anomalies such as aniridia or hemihypertrophy. CCSK has been found to be associated with a high rate of tumor relapse (even for stage I disease), and bone and brain metastases.[6,32] Initially, outcome was reported to be poor,[35] but, in the past few years with the utilization of both multidrug chemotherapy and abdominal radiotherapy, it has improved considerably.[4]

RHABDOID TUMOR OF THE KIDNEY

Rhabdoid tumor of the kidney (RTK), a highly-malignant tumor type, was identified in 1978.[14] Like CCSK, RTK is a monomorphous tumor. It is characterized by large uniform cells with abundant acidophilic cytoplasm (that often resembles that of

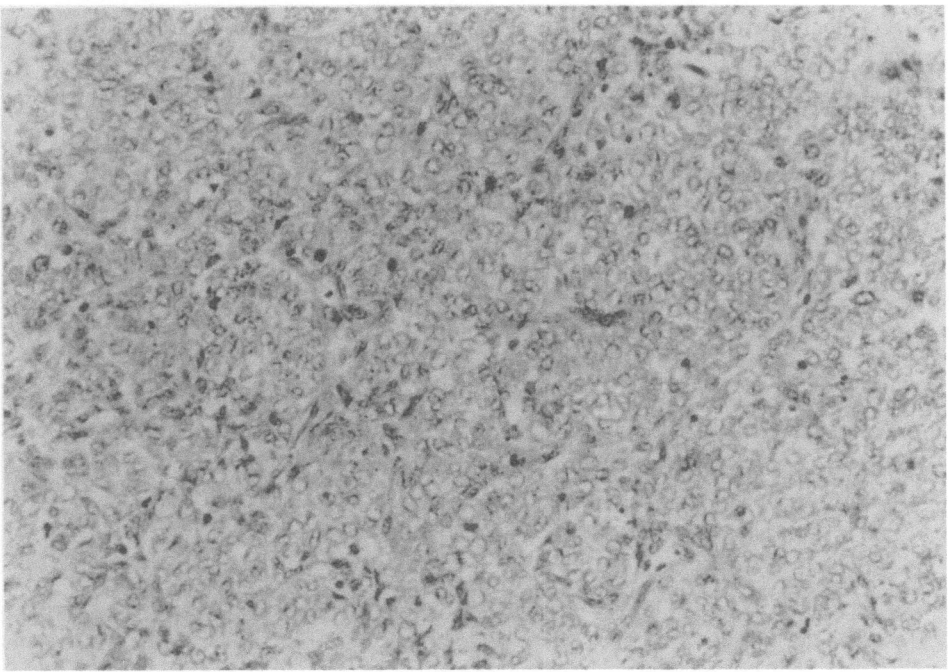

Fig. 2.6. Clear cell sarcoma of kidney (CCSK). This medium-magnification photograph shows the characteristic monomorphous appearance of CCSK, with pale-stained, polygonal tumor cells arranged in clusters separated by spindled septa. The polygonal cells have extremely pale nuclei and generally lack a clearly defined nucleolus. Courtesy of Dr. J. Bruce Beckwith, Department of Pathology, Loma Linda University, California. Reprinted with permission from M.J. Coppes, Wilms tumor: From cure to understanding, Critical Reviews in Oncology and Hematology 1995; 18:179-196. Copyright © Elsevier Scientific Publishers, Ireland Ltd.

myoblasts but is negative for markers of skeletal muscle), frequently containing a discrete zone of pale eosinophilia, and large nuclei having very prominent nucleoli (Fig. 2.7). This tumor is diagnosed in very young children, median age 13 months (range two months to five years), and is associated with high relapse rates (>80%) despite multimodality treatment.[36] It is occasionally a component of a multiple tumor syndrome.[37] The cell of origin for this tumor remains unknown.

CONCLUSIONS

Histopathologic analyses have identified several different tumor types among those previously aggregated under the classification of Wilms tumor. Meanwhile, Wilms tumors themselves have been subdivided into those with "favorable histology" and those with "anaplastic" features. Finally, it has now been recognized that the long-known precursor lesions can be subdivided into two types distinguished by their position within the renal lobe. The relative position within the lobe is a direct reflection of the chronology of development of the precursor lesion. PLNRs, found in the lobar periphery, develop later than ILNRs, which are found anywhere within the lobe. The morphological heterogeneity described probably reflects aberrant regulation of the same continuum of cell differentiation usually manifested by normal tissue counterparts. The more accurate histopathologic description of Wilms tumors and precursor lesions developed in the past years, has allowed us to start clarifying some of the molecular genetic events that determine different histopathologic phenotypes.

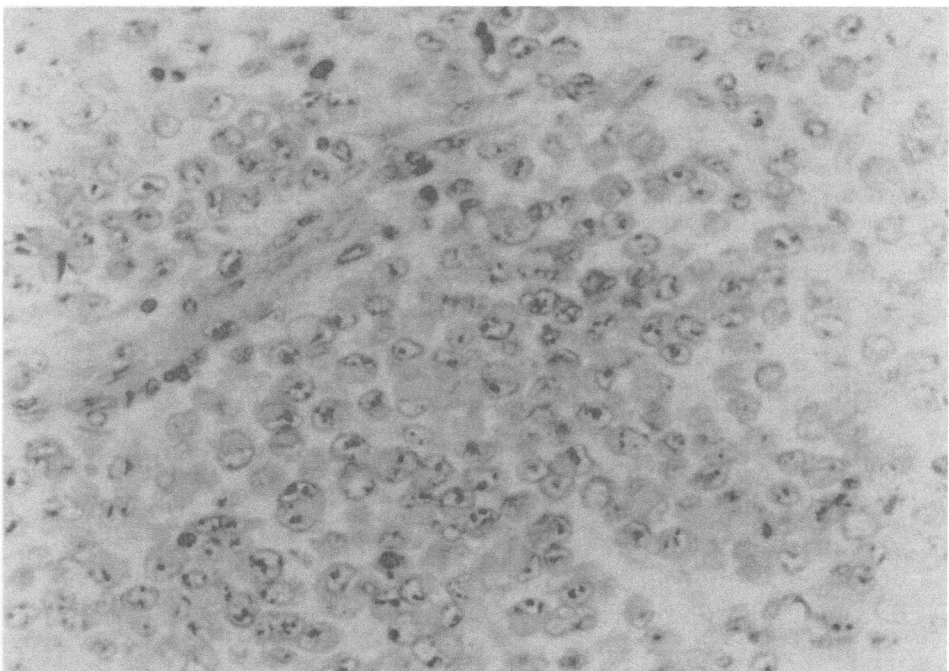

Fig. 2.7. Rhabdoid tumor of kidney (RTK). In this high-magnification view, the tumor cells are polygonal, with vesicular nuclei and a single large, darkly-stained nucleolus in each nucleus. Note the pale, globular cytoplasmic inclusions in most cells near the center of the field, often indenting nuclei. Courtesy of Dr. J. Bruce Beckwith, Department of Pathology, Loma Linda University, California. Reprinted with permission from M.J. Coppes, Wilms tumor: Reprinted with permission from M.J. Coppes, Wilms tumor: From cure to understanding, Critical Reviews in Oncology and Hematology 1995; 18:179-196. Copyright © Elsevier Scientific Publishers, Ireland Ltd.

REFERENCES

1. Eberth CJ: Myoma sarcomatodes renum. Virchows Arch 1872; 55:518-520.
2. Cohnheim J: Congenitales, quergestreiftes Muskelsarcom der Nieren. Virchows Arch Pathol Anat Physiol 1875; 65:64-69.
3. Wilms M: Die Mischgeschwülste der Niere. Leipzig: Verlag von Arthur Georgi, 1899:1-90.
4. Green DM, D'Angio GJ, Beckwith JB, Breslow N, Finklestein J, Kelalis P, Thomas P: Wilms' tumor (Nephroblastoma, renal embryoma). In Pizzo PA and Poplack DG (eds): Principles and Practice of Pediatric Oncology. Philadelphia: J.B. Lippincott Company, 1993:713-737.
5. Gonzalez-Crussi F: The pathology of Wilms' tumor. In: Gonzalez-Crussi F (eds): Wilms' Tumor (Nephroblastoma) and Related Renal Neoplasms of Childhood. Boca Raton, Florida: CRC Press, 1984:177-206.
6. Beckwith JB: Wilms' tumor and other renal tumors of childhood. In: Finegold M (eds): Pathology of Neoplasia in Children and Adolescents. Philadelphia: WB Saunders Company, 1986:313-332.
7. Mierau GW, Weeks DA, Beckwith JB: Ultrastructure and histogenesis of the renal tumors of childhood: An overview. Ultrastruct Pathol 1987; 11:313-333.
8. Altmannsberger M, Osborn M, Schäfer H, Schauer A, Weber K: Distinction of nephroblastomas from other childhood tumors using antibodies to intermediate filaments. Virchows Archiv B 1984; 45:113-124.
9. Lawler W, Marsden HB, Palmer ML: Wilms' tumor-histologic variations and prognosis. Cancer 1975; 40:1122-1126.
10. Chatten J: Epithelial differentiation in Wilms' tumor: A clinicopathologic appraisal. Perspect Pediatr Pathol 1976; 3:225-254.
11. Chambers CH, Camitta BM, Tang TT, McCreadie SR: Nephroblastoma (Wilms' tumor): Tubule density and prognosis. Med Pediatr Oncol 1978; 5:127-135.
12. Beckwith JB: Grading pediatric tumors. Care of the child with cancer. New York: American Cancer Society, 1979:39-44.
13. Bonadio JF, Storer B, Norkool P, Farewell VT, Beckwith JB, D'Angio GJ: Anaplastic Wilms' tumor: clinical and pathological studies. J Clin Oncol 1985; 3:513-520.
14. Beckwith JB, Palmer NF: Histopathology and prognosis of Wilms' tumor. Results from the first National Wilms' Tumor Study. Cancer 1978; 41:1937-1948.
15. Delemarre JFM, Sandstedt B, Gérard-Marchant R, Tournade MF. SIOP nephroblastoma trials and studies, morphological aspects. In the proceedings of the 13th meeting of the International Society of Paediatric Oncology, September 15-19, 1981. Mareseille: Exerpta Medica, 1982.

16. Zuppan CW, Beckwith JB, Luckey DW: Anaplasia in unilateral Wilms' tumor: A report from the National Wilms' Tumor Study Pathology Center. Human Pathol 1988; 19:1199-209.

17. Faria P, Beckwith JB: A new definition of focal anaplasia (FA) in Wilms tumor (WT) identifies cases with good outcome. A report from the National Wilms tumor Study. Mod Pathol 1993; 6:3p.

18. Bennington JL, Beckwith J: Tumors of the kidney, renal pelvis, and ureter (Fasc.12). In Atlas of tumor pathology. Washington, DC: Armed Forces Institute of Pathology, 1975.

19. Bove KE, McAdams AJ: The nephroblastomatosis complex and its relationship to Wilms' tumor: A clinicopathologic treatise. Perspect Pediatr Pathol 1976; 3:185-223.

20. Beckwith JB, Kiviat NB, Bonadio JF: Nephrogenic rests, nephroblastomatosis, and the pathogenesis of Wilms' tumor. Pediatr Pathol 1990; 10:1-36.

21. Fine H: The developments of the lobes of the metanephros and fetal kidney. Acta Anat (Basel) 1982; 113:93-107.

22. Inke G: The protolobar structure of the human kidney: Its biologic and clinical significance. New York: Alan R Liss, 1988.

23. Beckwith JB: Precursor lesions of Wilms tumor: clinical and biological implications. Med Pediatr Oncol 1993; 21:158-168.

24. Park S, Bernard A, Bove KE, Sens DA, Hazen-Martin DJ, Garvin HA, Haber DA: Inactivation of *WT1* in nephrogenic rests, genetic precursors to Wilms' tumour. Nature Genetics 1993; 5:363-367.

25. Bolande RP, Brough AJ, Izant RJ: Congenital mesoblastic nephroma of infants. A report of eight cases and the relationship to Wilms' tumor. Pediatrics 1976; 40:272-278.

26. Howell CG, Othersen HB, Kiviat NE, Norkool P, Beckwith JB, D'Angio GJ: Therapy and outcome in 51 children with mesoblastic nephroma: A report of the National Wilms' Tumor Study. J Pediatr Surg 1982; 17:826-831.

27. Sandstedt BE, Delemarre JFM, Krul EJ, Tournade MF: Mesoblastic nephromas: A study of 29 tumours from the SIOP nephroblastoma file. Histopathology 1985; 9:741-750.

28. Beckwith JB, Kiviat NB: Multilocular renal cysts and cystic renal tumors. Am J Roentgenol 1981; 136:435-436.

29. Snyder HM, Lack E, Chetty-Baktavizion S, Brauer SB, Colodna AM, Retik AB: Congenital mesoblastic nephroma: Relationship to other renal tumors in infancy. J Urol 1981; 126:513-516.

30. Coppes MJ, Bonetta L, Huang A, Hoban P, Chilton-MacNeill S, Campbell CE, Weksberg R, Yeger H, Reeve AE, Williams BRG: Loss of heterozygosity mapping in Wilms tumor indicates the involvement of three distinct regions and a limited role for non-disjunction or mitotic recombination. Genes Chrom Cancer 1992; 5:326-334.

31. Tomlinson GE, Argyle JC, Velasco S, Nisen PD: Molecualr characterization of congenital mesoblastic nephroma and its distinction from Wilms tumor. Cancer 1992; 70:2358-2361.

32. Kidd JM: Exclusion of certain renal neoplasms from the category of Wilms' tumor. Am J Pathol 1970; 59:16a.

33. Marsden HB, Lawler W, Kumar PM: Bone metastazing renal tumor of childhood. Morphological and clinical features, and differences from Wilms' tumor. Cancer 1978; 42:1922-1928.

34. Sandstedt BE, Delemarre JFM, Harms D, Tournade MF: Sarcomatous Wilms' tumour with clear cells and hyalinization. A study of 38 tumours in children from the SIOP nephroblastoma file. Histopathology 1987; 9:273-285.

35. Haas JE, Bonadio JF, Beckwith JB: Clear cell sarcoma of the kidney with emphasis on ultrastructural studies. Cancer 1984; 54:2978-2987.

36. Stassinopolou A, Tournade MF, Ducourtieux M, Terrier-Lacombe MJ, Habrand JL, Gruner M, Valteau-Couanet D, Lemerle J: The malignant rhabdoid tumor (MRT) of the kidney: A rare but unsolved problem. Med and Pediatr Oncol 1991; 19:389.

37. Palmer NF, Sutow W: Clinical aspects of the rhabdoid tumor of the kidney: A report from the National Wilms' Tumor Study Group. Med Pediatr Oncol 1983; 11:242-245.

CHAPTER 3

GENETICS OF WILMS TUMOR

INTRODUCTION

Most Wilms tumors are unilateral and sporadic, but approximately 5-10% are bilateral[1] and a further 1-2% show familial recurrence.[2,3] The observation that Wilms tumor, like retinoblastoma (a childhood tumor of the retina), can be unilateral or bilateral at presentation, has been of particular interest in view of Knudson and Strong's proposed two-hit model for the development of certain cancers. In 1971, Knudson compared the incidence of unilateral versus multiple retinoblastomas in children with a positive family history and subsequently calculated the number of events required for tumor development.[4] Based on the Poisson distribution for rare events, he predicted that retinoblastoma develops as a consequence of two rate-limiting cellular events.[4] A year later, a similar model was put forward for the development of Wilms tumor.[5] This hypothesis predicts that most or all Wilms tumors will contain either one or two mutant Wilms tumor suppressor allelles and no wild-type allele. The first hit referred to in the two-hit hypothesis will result in a mutation in one Wilms tumor suppressor allele. The cell undergoing this mutation will still be phenotypically normal but will be predisposed to tumor initiation following a second hit. The number of mutant alleles in the tumor will depend upon whether the second hit, which results in loss of the wild-type allele, occurs through chromosome loss, non disjunction, mitotic recombination or a second mutation (Fig. 3.1).

The "two-hit" hypothesis suggests that there are heritable and non-heritable forms of cancer. In the heritable* form, the first cellular

---

*Heritable Wilms tumor should not be confused with familial Wilms tumor. Unlike retinoblastoma, only 1-2% of Wilms tumors are familial. Siblings of an affected child with heritable Wilms tumor are, in the large majority of cases, not at increased risk of developing Wilms tumor, as the germline mutation usually occurs de novo and therefore is not inherited from an affected parent.

Wilms Tumor: Clinical and Molecular Characterization, by Max J. Coppes, Christine E. Campbell, and Bryan R.G. Williams. © 1995 R.G. Landes Company.

event is prezygotic, leading to a constitutional or germline mutation that will be present in all cells of the resultant embryo. A
single second event in any one cell of a susceptible target tissue
(retina or kidney, for example) will lead to tumor development.
The model predicts that individuals who carry a germline mutation are not only at risk of developing multiple tumors, since all
the cells will carry the first event and only one additional event is
required to allow tumorigenesis, but also that these individuals will

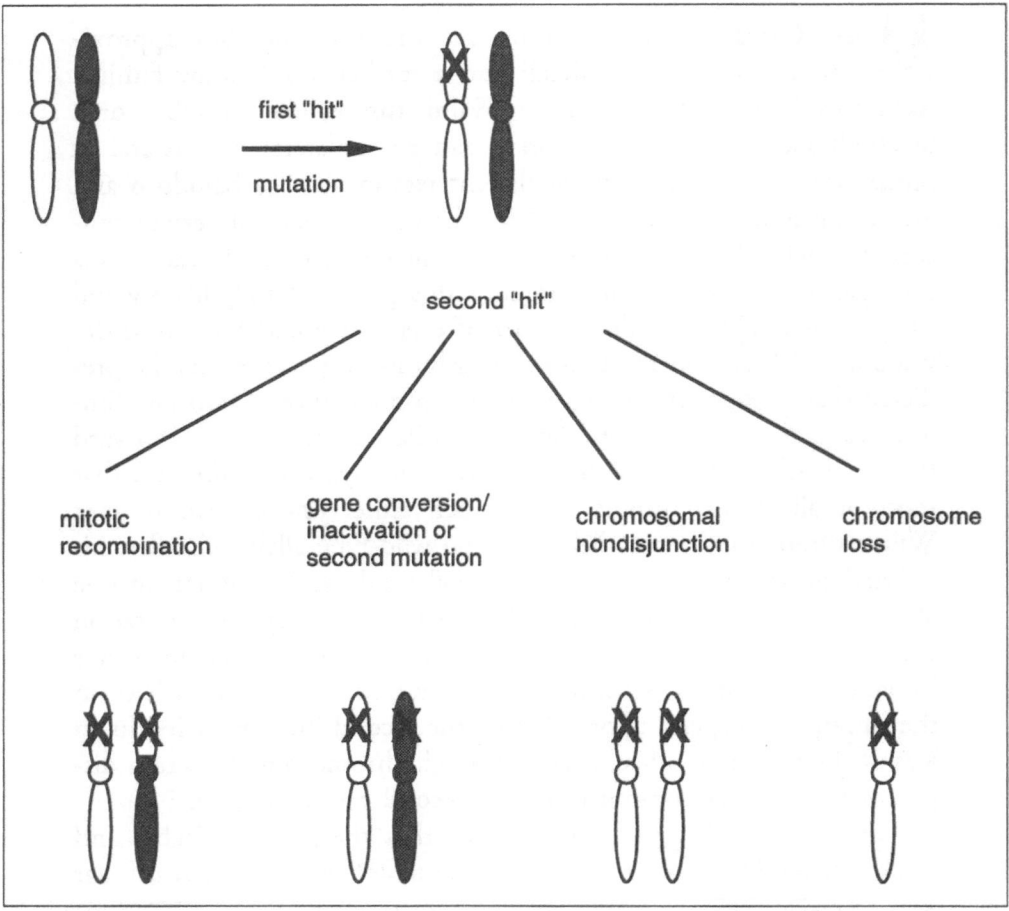

Fig. 3.1. Mechanisms leading to phenotypic expression of a recessive WT1 mutation. The first "hit"
involves a mutation that inactivates one WT1 allele. The second "hit" can involve mitotic recombination
which will lead to a loss of heterozygosity for all genes distal to the recombination event. A second
mechanism involves gene conversion/ inactivation or a second mutation which will affect only the WT1
gene. Chromosome nondisjunction will result in two copies of the chromosome carrying the mutation
while chromosome loss will result in a single copy of the mutant chromosome.

acquire their tumor at a relatively early age compared to those who do not carry a germline mutation. By contrast, in the non-hereditary tumors, which also require two cellular events, both mutational events must occur within the same somatic cell lineage in order to cause a tumor. Because the probability of this happening in more than one cell is small, these individuals are unlikely to develop more than one tumor. Similarly, non-hereditary (usually unilateral) tumors are expected to develop at a later age than hereditary Wilms tumors.

The two-hit hypothesis has been confirmed at the molecular level for retinoblastoma.[6] The isolation of *RB1*, the retinoblastoma susceptibility gene, mapping to chromosome 13q14,[7,8] led subsequently to examples of families segregating retinoblastoma in which transmission of a mutant *RB1* allele to each of the affected individuals (first hit) was followed by loss of the wild-type (normal) *RB1* allele in the tumor (second hit).[9] Likewise, tumors harboring two different somatic *RB1* mutations or deletions were also described (reviewed in ref. 9)

The genetic events leading to the development of Wilms tumor, however, have turned out to be more complex, despite early loss of heterozygosity (LOH) data that seemed to favor a genetic model very similar to the one described for retinoblastoma. It is now clear that several loci are involved: one at 11p13, one at 11p15, one at 16q, possibly one at 1p and finally an as yet unidentified "familial locus."[10] The identification of each of these loci resulted from a combination of clinical observations, karyotype analyses and molecular genetic studies. Much of this work has been based on the evaluation of patients who develop Wilms tumor in association with a number of rare congenital anomalies, including aniridia, the WAGR syndrome, hemihypertrophy and the BWS.

CYTOGENETICS

Children with Wilms tumor, aniridia, genitourinary malformations, and mental retardation, referred to by the acronym WAGR syndrome, carry specific cytogenetic anomalies which have been instrumental in the cloning of *WT1*, one of the Wilms tumor suppressor genes. Chromosomal studies using high-resolution banding techniques allowed the identification of chromosomal regions within individual chromosomes and demonstrated that children with

with WAGR carry interstitial deletions within the short arm of one copy of chromosome 11,[11] at band p13.[12] That the constitutional 11p13 deletion observed in patients with the WAGR syndrome is directly related to Wilms tumor predisposition was strengthened by observations of 11p13 deletions in Wilms tumor cells from patients with Wilms tumor and normal constitutional chromosomes.[13,14] Segregation of a translocation disrupting 11p13 with aniridia in two families with hereditary aniridia,[15,16] in whom the affected individuals did not develop Wilms tumor, suggested that the putative Wilms tumor gene was distinct from the aniridia gene. Genitourinary malformations, on the other hand, appear to be more closely linked to Wilms tumor. Indeed, it is now known that the WAGR deletion encompasses a number of contiguous genes, including the aniridia gene *PAX6* and the Wilms tumor suppressor gene *WT1*. Loss of one copy of the *PAX6* gene is responsible for aniridia,[17] while loss of one *WT1* allele may confer genitourinary defects in addition to constituting the first hit required for the development of Wilms tumor (see chapter 7).

Following the first cytogenetic studies of sporadic Wilms tumor,[13,14] there have been over 150 additional karyotypes, of which approximately 60% were abnormal.[18] In 1992, Slater and Mannens published a comprehensive study of the cytogenetic changes occurring in Wilms tumor.[18] They demonstrated that in general chromosome gains are far more common than chromosome losses, particularly involving the C-group chromosomes and chromosomes 13, 17, 18 and 20.[18] Of these, trisomy 12 is especially prevalent. Not surprisingly, changes involving the short arm of chromosome 11, which have been reported in approximately 25% of all Wilms tumors, were the most common structural karyotypic alterations noted. In addition, there was preferential loss of the short and long arms of chromosome 1 and the long arm of chromosome 16 (especially involving bands 16q11 and 16q13).[18] Changes in the short arm of chromosome 1 have also been reported in other pediatric maligancies, including neuroblastoma, retinoblastoma and rhabdomyosarcoma,[19] while certain changes on chromosome 16q have been reported in Ewing sarcoma, peripheral neuroectodermal tumors, uterine cancer and rhabdomyosarcoma.[18] The fact that these changes occur in so many tumors suggests that the genetic alterations on chromosomes 1 and 16q are likely secondary events and associated with tumor progression rather than tumor initiation.

LOSS OF HETEROZYGOSITY

In tumors resulting from recessive mutations, both alleles of the tumor suppressor gene are inactivated in sequence, the first one by mutation and the second frequently by somatic recombination or nondisjunction. Consequently, loss of heterozygosity (LOH) is frequently observed in these tumors. Because LOH for polymorphic markers reflects the role of allele loss in the development of such tumors, LOH studies have been useful in detecting and localizing tumor suppressor genes. The first LOH studies in Wilms tumor were performed with DNA probes mapping to the short arm of chromosome 11.[20-23] While these probes were de facto restricted to the 11p15 region, the demonstrated LOH was interpreted to include chromosome 11p13, since this region had previously been shown to carry cytogenetic deletions in patients with the WAGR syndrome, i.e. children with an increased risk for the development of Wilms tumor. Therefore, it was assumed that LOH for 11p15 markers would also reflect LOH for the 11p13 region. Consequently, these early data were interpreted as additional evidence supporting the presence of a tumor suppressor gene for Wilms tumor at 11p13. However, in a subset of Wilms tumors, LOH is indeed restricted to chromosome 11p15, with maintenance of heterozygosity for markers at chromosome 11p13.[24-29] This observation suggests the existence of a second independent Wilms tumor suppressor locus on the short arm of chromosome 11, at 11p15. Although the gene has not been cloned it has been given the designation *WT2* (see chapter 8).

In the past two years, it has become evident that tumor specific LOH for markers at chromosome 16q occurs in approximately 20% of patients with Wilms tumor,[29-31] while LOH for chromosome 1p markers has been demonstrated in about 12% of cases studied.[31] As mentioned earlier several tumors exhibit LOH for these chromosomal regions, suggesting that LOH for 16q and 1p may be associated with tumor progression. Indeed, it has recently been reported that LOH for chromosome 16q markers in Wilms tumor correlates with an adverse outcome.[31] The difference in relapse-free survival for those with, compared to those without, LOH for 16q markers remained significant when adjusted for histology or for stage.[31] The correlation between LOH for chromosome 1p markers and outcome showed a trend (p=0.08), but the sample size was too small to establish statistical significance. These data suggest that the underlying genetic events associated with LOH for chromosome 16q and possibly 1p genes in Wilms tumor are involved with tumor progression rather than tumor development. This is consistent with the fact that, thus far, no association has been reported between constitutional deletions at 16q or 1p and an increased risk of Wilms tumor.

THE 11p13 LOCUS

The association between sporadic aniridia and Wilms tumor was the first observation that ultimately lead to the cloning and characterization of *WT1*, the Wilms tumor suppressor gene at chromosome 11p13 (see chapter 4). It is now clear that aniridia and Wilms tumor constitute a "contiguous gene syndrome" in which deletion of adjacent genes can result in a combination of congenital anomalies. Further support for the existence of a tumor suppressor gene at 11p13 was derived from studies demonstrating tumor specific LOH for chromosome 11p. Subsequently, a series of hybrid mapping panels established from patients with constitutional deletions further defined the region of interest. Physical maps spanning the region from the catalase (*CAT*) and β follicle stimulating hormone (*FSHβ*), genes that flank the WAGR locus, were established using newly cloned DNA sequences and deletions or balanced chromosomal abnormalities associated with one or multiple features of the WAGR syndrome. Ultimately, a case of a sporadic unilateral Wilms tumor, referred to as WiT-13, with an apparently normal karyotype, that nonetheless demonstrated a homozygous deletion for D11S87, a random DNA fragment mapping between the *CAT* locus and the *FSHβ* locus, established the physical boundaries within which the Wilms tumor gene at 11p13 had to lie.[32] Molecular analyses of the DNA mapping to this region led to the identification of *WT1*,[33-35] as described in more detail in the next chapter. Also, we reported a second transcript, *WIT1*, transcribed in divergent direction from *WT1*.[35,36] Whether or not *WIT1* encodes a functional polypeptide remains to be determined (see chapter 4).

THE 11p15 LOCUS

As discussed earlier, LOH was demonstrated in a subset of tumors for markers telomeric of 11p13,[24-29] suggesting the existence of a second Wilms tumor suppressor locus on the short arm of chromosome 11, at 11p15. This second putative Wilms tumor suppressor gene has already been designated *WT2*. A second tumor suppressor gene at 11p15 may explain the association of Wilms tumor with the BWS. BWS is characterized by numerous growth abnormalities and a predisposition to several neoplasms, including Wilms tumor, adrenocortical carcinoma, hepatoblastoma, rhabdomyosarcoma and occasionally pancreatic tumors and neuroblastoma.[37]

Although most BWS cases are sporadic, approximately 15% are familial or found in association with chromosomal abnormalities.[38] Because the clinical findings are variable and tend to become less obvious with age, it is suspected that many adults with this syndrome are not diagnosed. As a consequence, familial inheritance may be masked. Familial BWS is transmitted as an autosomal dominant disease with reduced penetrance and variable ex-pressivity.[39] Moreover, genomic imprinting most likely accounts for the unusual patterns of transmission described in some families. Linkage analysis revealed that the locus for the familial form maps to chromosome 11p15.[40,41] Additional evidence for the involvement of chromosome 11p15 in BWS was provided by the demonstration of constitutional cytogenetic anomalies exclusively involving 11p15 in patients with sporadic BWS.[42,43] The abnormalities observed usually involved duplication of chromosome 11p15 and, interestingly, in all informative cases, the duplicated chromosomal segment has been of paternal origin.[42-49] A sex-dependent mode of transmission in this syndrome was also found in the described BWS patients with uniparental paternal disomy for chromosome 11, all whom have been shown to carry two copies of the paternal chromosome 11 and consequently no maternal chromosome 11.[50,51]

Whether or not the BWS gene and the *WT2* gene are the same or two separate but closely-linked genes is unclear. However, the mechanisms leading to BWS and Wilms tumor seem to be dissimilar. LOH data clearly suggest that Wilms tumor results from homozygous inactivation of the putative *WT2* gene, similar to the inactivation of *WT1* in certain Wilms tumors[52] or *RB1* in retinoblastoma,[9] while the BWS seems to result from the presence of two paternal copies of the BWS gene. Therefore, it is still unclear whether this region harbors two distinct genes with different roles or a single gene that under different conditions acts either as a growth promoter (BWS) or tumor suppressor (Wilms tumor).

GENOMIC IMPRINTING

As discussed above, early chromosome 11p LOH data revealed that allele loss was not a random event, as previously suggested by Knudson, but that the maternal allele was preferentially lost.[21,22,53] In an attempt to provide a model that would explain the observed preferential retention of the paternal allele, Wilkins proposed a role for genomic imprinting in Wilms tumorigenesis.[54] The term imprinting refers to the marking of genetic information at the chromosomal level, distinguishing maternally from paternally-derived genetic alleles. A role for imprinting has been suggested in the phenotypic expression of several genetic disorders and in the explanation of traits and conditions that do not show Mendelian inheritance patterns. Evidence for the existence of genomic imprinting comes from several observations which have been reviewed elsewhere[55-58] and are discussed further in chapter 8.

Based on the similarity of known genomically imprinted genes and the regulatory genes of the two-hit model (both are expressed at certain stages, both have to be switched on and off), Wilkins proposed that a maternally-derived transforming gene (T_R) closely linked to the recessive Wilms tumor gene on chromosome 11 is imprinted (Fig. 3.2).[54] The paternal and maternal Wilms tumor gene can both be expressed in the embryo, but the maternal T_R gene is rendered inactive by a genomic imprinting event (e.g., methylation). The first hit, from the two-hit model, can be on either chromosome and, if the second hit is a localized mutation, inactivation of the Wilms tumor gene product derepresses the T_R gene and results in the development of a tumor. If the second hit involves mitotic recombination, rather than a localized mutation, resulting in the loss of a larger region or all of the chromosome, the T_R gene will be fully expressed only if the paternal chromosome 11 is retained. Implicit in this model is the assumption that one of the T_R genes controlled by the Wilms tumor gene should be on chromosome 11. An alternative explanation, which does not involve a T_R gene, was suggested by Reik and Surani,[59] based on a suggestion made by Sapienza and colleagues (Fig. 3.3).[60] This hypothesis states that the first mutation in the Wilms tumor gene on chromosome 11 occurs on the

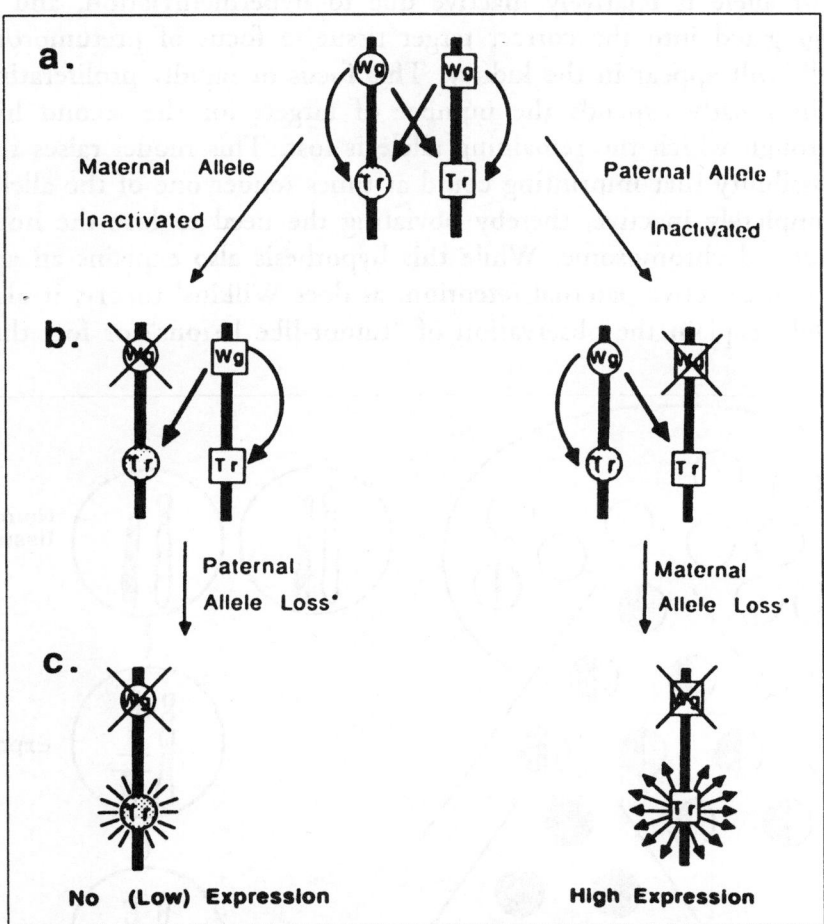

Fig. 3.2. Model proposed by R. Wilkins to explain the bias to tumor specific retention of the paternal allele. A) In normal cells the two alleles of a transforming gene (T_R) are kept in a suppressed state by the diffusable product (arrowed) of the two Wilms regulatory gene alleles (Wg). B) If one Wg allele is rendered inactive (through either somatic mutation in sporadic Wilms or inheritance in familial Wilms), suppression of T_R genes still continues irrespective of whether the paternal (unshaded square) or maternal (unshaded circle) alleles are involved. C) When the second Wg gene is lost, the T_R genes are released from the suppressed state and are expressed at a high level (if not imprinted) or a low level or not at all (if imprinted). In the model shown the maternal allele is imprinted (shaded circle). From Richard J. Wilkins, Genomic imprinting and carcinogenesis, Lancet 1:329-331. Copyright © The Lancet Ltd., 1988. The fundamental mechanisms involved in imprinting remain to be elucidated.

paternal allele in embryonic cells where the maternal Wilms tumor allele is relatively inactive due to hypermethylation, and if segregated into the correct target tissue, a focus of pretumorous cells will appear in the kidney. This focus of rapidly proliferating cells greatly expands the number of targets for the second hit, through which the remaining allele is lost. This model raises the possibility that imprinting could at times render one of the alleles completely inactive, thereby obviating the need to lose the non-mutated chromosome. While this hypothesis also explains an apparent selective paternal retention, as does Wilkins' theory, it also could explain the observation of "tumor-like lesions" or foci that

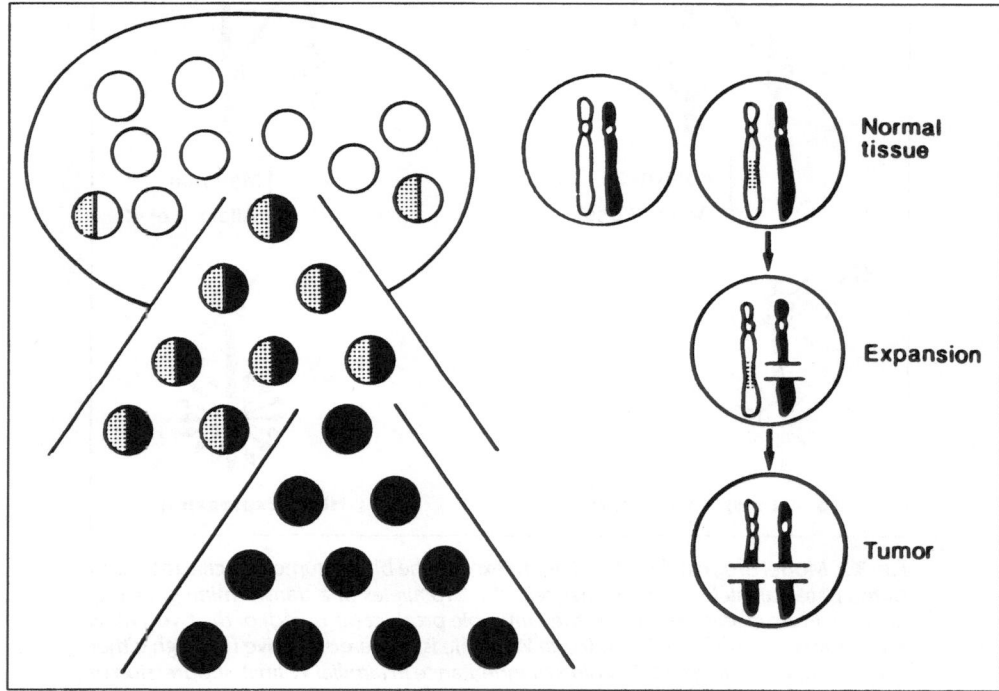

Fig. 3.3. Model proposed by Reik to explain the preferential loss of the maternal allele in tumors. Most cells in the target tissue have maternal (open) and paternal (filled) chromosomes, both of which express either the RB or the Wilms tumor gene. On some maternal chromosomes, however, these genes are repressed by imprinting (stippled area). If the first mutation happens to be on a paternal chromosome opposite the relatively inactive maternal allele, this population of cells will expand. This expansion will neither occur with the first hit on a paternal chromosome opposite an active maternal nor with the first hit on a maternal chromosome. The expanded population now represents a much increased target for the second event — loss of the maternal allele (by somatic recombination in this case). Note that if the second mutation does not occur, the initial focus of growth may not progress into a tumor. Reprinted with permission from Nature, 338:112-113. Copyright © 1989 Macmillan Magazines Limited.

seem to have regressed in several tissues, including kidneys. Imprinting is discussed further in chapter 8.

THE FAMILIAL WILMS TUMOR LOCUS

The low incidence of familial Wilms tumor (1-2.5% of all cases), has complicated the search for a gene involved in familial Wilms tumor. Multi-point linkage analysis studies have excluded both the 11p13 and 11p15 loci in three pedigrees,[61,62] and chromosome 11p13 only in another pedigree,[63] as loci involved in familial Wilms tumor. Of interest is the observation that, in one affected member of one the four pedigrees, 11p15 LOH was demonstrated.[61] However, the allele retained in the tumor was shown to be inherited from the unaffected father, a result inconsistent with the unmasking of an inherited recessive defect at 11p15.

The description of a transmitted single nucleotide deletion within *WT1* from father to son, both of whom had Wilms tumor,[64] suggests the involvement of chromosome 11p13 in one case of familial Wilms tumor. Detailed analysis of additional familial Wilms tumor cases will need to be performed in order to determine if *WT1* mutations are responsible for additional familial cases.

CONCLUSIONS

The introduction of the two-hit hypothesis in 1971 by Knudson suggested that only a small number of genetic events, of which two are rate-limiting, are necessary for the transformation of a normal cell into a cancer cell. The observation of a heterozygous constitutional deletion in patients with the WAGR syndrome identified chromosome 11p13 as a region of interest in the development of Wilms tumor. Subsequently other chromosome areas have been implicated (11p15, 16q, 1p, the unknown "familial" locus) in Wilms tumor, revealing a more complex mechanism than initially expected. One Wilms tumor susceptibility gene, *WT1* mapping to 11p13, has been cloned and characterized (see chapter 4). Current data suggest that this gene plays an important role in urogenital development (see chapter 5) and in the development of certain Wilms tumors (see chapter 7). Understanding the role of all the different Wilms tumor loci will require the isolation and characterization of the specific genes that they encode. Potential interactions between these genes are suggested by the presence within individual Wilms tumors of molecular lesions affecting more than one locus.[26,65]

References

1. Coppes MJ, De Kraker J, Van Dijken PJ, Perry HJ, Delemarre JF, Tournade MF, Lemerle J, Voûte PA: Bilateral Wilms' tumor: Long-term survival and some epidemiological features. J Clin Oncol 1989; 7:310-315.

2. Breslow NE, Beckwith JB: Epidemiological features of Wilms' tumor: Results of the National Wilms' Tumor Study. J Natl Cancer Inst 1982; 68:429-436.

3. Bonaïti-Pellié C, Chompret A, Tournade MF, Hochez J, Moutou C, Zucker JM, Roché H, Tron P, Frappaz D, Munzer M, Bachelot C, Dusol F, Sommelet-Olive D, Lemerle J: Genetics and epidemiology of Wilms' tumor: The French Wilms' Tumor Study. Med Pediatr Oncol 1992; 20:284-291.

4. Knudson AG: Mutation and cancer: Statistical study of retinoblastoma. Proc Natl Acad Sci USA 1971; 68:820-823.

5. Knudson AG, Strong LC: Mutation and cancer: A model for Wilms' tumor of kidney. J Natl Cancer Inst 1972; 48:313-324.

6. Hamel PA, Phillips RA, Muncaster M, Gallie BL: Speculations on the roles of RB1 in tissue specific differentiation, tumor initiation, and tumor progression. FASEB J 1993; 7:846-854.

7. Friend SH, Bernards R, Rogelj S, Weinberg RA, Rapaport JM, Albert DM, Drye TP: A human DNA segment with properties of the gene that predisposes to retinoblastoma and osteosarcoma. Nature 1986; 323:643-646.

8. Lee WH, Bookstein R, Hong F, Young LJ, Shew Y, Lee EY: Human retinoblastoma susceptibility gene: cloning, identification, and sequence. Science 1987; 253:1394-9.

9. Gallie B, Squire J, Goddard A, Dunn JM, Canton M, Hinton D, Zhu X, Phillips RA: Mechanism of oncogenesis in retinoblastoma. Lab Invest 1990; 62:394-408.

10. Coppes MJ, Williams BRG: The molecular genetics of Wilms tumor. Cancer Invest 1994; 12:57-65.

11. Riccardi VM, Sujansky E, Smith AC, Francke U: Chromosomal imbalance in the aniridia-Wilms' tumor association: 11p interstitial deletion. Pediatrics 1978; 61:604-610.

12. Riccardi VM, Hittner HM, Francke U, Yunis JJ, Ledbetter D, Borges W: The aniridia-Wilms tumor association: The critical role of chromosome band 11p13. Cancer Genet Cytogenet 1980; 2:131-137.

13. Kaneko Y, Egues MC, Rowley JD: Interstitial deletion of the short arm of chromosome 11 limited to Wilms tumor cells in a patient without aniridia. Cancer Res 1981; 41:4577-4578.

14. Slater RM, De Kraker J: Chromosome number 11 and Wilms tumor. Cancer Genet Cytogenet 1982; 5:237-245.

15. Simola KO, Knuutila S, Kaitila I, Pirkola A, Pohja P: Familial aniridia and translocation t(4;1)(q22-p13) without Wilms tumor. Hum Genet 1983; 63:158-161.

16. Moore JW, Hyman S, Antonarakis SE, Mules EH, Thomas GH: Hum Genet 1986; 72:297-302.

17. Ton CCT, Hirvonen H, Miwa H, Weil MM, Monaghan P, Jordan T, Van Heyningen V, Hastie ND, Meijers-Heijboer H, Drechsler M, Royer-Pokora B, Cllins F, Swaroop A, Strong LC, Saunders GF: Positional cloning and characterization of a paired box- and homeobox-containing gene from the aniridia region. Cell 1991; 67:1059-1074.

18. Slater RM, Mannens MMAM: Cytogenetics and Molecular Genetics of Wilms' tumor of childhood. Cancer Genet Cytogenet 1992; 61:111-121.

19. Douglass EC, Green AA, Hayes FA, Etcubanas E, Horowitz M, Wiliminas JA: Chromosome 1 abnormalities: A common feature of pediatric solid tumors. J Natl Cancer Inst 1985; 75:51-54.

20. Koufos A, Hansen MF, Lampkin BC, Workman ML, Copeland NG, Jenkins NA, Cavenee WK: Loss of alleles at loci on human chromosome 11 during genesis of Wilms' tumour. Nature 1984; 309:170-172.

21. Orkin SH, Goldman DS Sallan, S.E.: Development of homozygosity for chromosome 11p markers in Wilms' tumour. Nature 1984; 309:172-4.

22. Reeve AE, Housiaux PJ, Gardner RJM, Chewings WE, Grindley RM, Millow LJ: Loss of a Harvey ras allele in sporadic Wilms' tumour. Nature 1984; 309:174-6.

23. Fearon ER, Vogelstein B, Feinberg AP: Somatic deletion and duplication of genes on chromosome 11 in Wilms' tumours. Nature 1984; 309:176-178.

24. Mannens M, Slater RM, Heyting C, Bliek J, de KJ, Coad N, de P, Holthuizen P, Pearson PL: Molecular nature of genetic changes resulting in loss of heterozygosity of chromosome 11 in Wilms' tumours. Hum Genet 1988; 81:41-8.

25. Reeve AE, Sih SA, Raizis AM, Feinberg AP: Loss of allelic heterozygosity at a second locus on chromosome 11 in sporadic Wilms' tumor cells. Molec Cell Biol 1989; 9:1799-1803.

26. Henry I, Grandjouan S, Couillin P, Barichard F, Huerre-Jeanpierre C, Glaser T, Philip T, Lenoir G, Chaussain JL, Junien C: Tumor-specific loss of 11p15.5 alleles in del11p13 Wilms tumor and in familial adrenocortical carcinoma. Proc Natl Acad Sci USA 1989; 86:3247-3251.

27. Mannens M, Devilee P, Bliek J, Mandjes I, de Kraker J, Heyting C, Slater RM, Westerveld A: Loss of heterozygosity in Wilms' tumors, studied for six putative tumor suppressor regions, is limited to chromosome 11. Cancer Res 1990; 50:3279-3283.

28. Wadey RB, Pal N, Buckle B, Yeomans E, Pritchard J, Cowell JK: Loss of heterozygosity in Wilms' tumour involves two distinct regions of chromosome 11. Oncogene 1990; 5:901-7.

29. Coppes MJ, Bonetta L, Huang A, Hoban P, Chilton-MacNeill S, Campbell CE, Weksberg R, Yeger H, Reeve AE, Williams BRG: Loss of heterozygosity mapping in Wilms tumor indicates the involvement of three distinct regions and a limited role for non-disjunction or mitotic recombination. Genes Chrom Cancer 1992; 5:326-334.

30. Maw MA, Grundy PE, Millow LJ, Eccles MR, Dunn RS, Smith PJ, Feinberg AP, Law DJ, Paterson MC, Telzerow PE, Callen DF, Thompson AD, Richards RI, Reeve AE: A third Wilms' tumor locus on chromosome 16q. Cancer Res 1992; 52:3094-3098.

31. Grundy PE, Telzerow PE, Breslow N, Moskess J, Huff V, Paterson MC: Loss of heterozygosity for chromosomes 16q and 1p in Wilms' tumors predicts an adverse outcome. Cancer Res 1994; 54:2331-2333.

32. Lewis WH, Yeger H, Bonetta L, Chan HLS, Kang J, Junien C, Cowell J, Jones C, Dafoe LA: Homozygous deletion of a DNA marker from chromosome 11p13 in sporadic Wilms tumor. Genomics 1988; 3:25-31.

33. Call KM, Glaser T, Ito CY, Buckler AJ, Pelletier J, Haber DA, Rose EA, Kral A, Yeger H, Lewis WH, Jones C, Housman DE: Isolation and characterization of a zinc finger polypeptide gene at the human chromosome 11 Wilms' tumor locus. Cell 1990; 60:509-520.

34. Gessler M, Poustka A, Cavenee W, Neve RL, Orkin SH, Bruns GA: Homozygous deletion in Wilms tumours of a zinc-finger gene identified by chromosome jumping. Nature 1990; 343:774-778.

35. Bonetta L, Kuehn SE, Huang A, Law DJ, Kalikin LM, Koi M, Reeve AE, Brownstein BH, Yeger H, Williams BRG, Feinberg AP: Wilms tumor locus on 11p13 defined by multiple CpG island-associated transcripts. Science 1990; 250:994-997.

36. Huang A, Campbell CE, Bonetta L, McAndrews -Hill M, Chilton-MacNeill S, Coppes MJ, Law DJ, Feinberg AP, Yeger H, Williams BRG: Tissue, developmental, and tumor-specific expression of divergent transcripts in Wilms tumor. Science 1990; 250:991-994.

37. Wiedemann H-R: Tumours and hemihypertrophy associated with Wiedemann-Beckwith syndrome. Eur J Pediatr 1983; 141:129.

38. Pettenati MJ, Haines JL, Higgins RR, Wappner RS, Palmer CG, Weaver DD: Wiedemann-Beckwith syndrome: Presentation of clinical and cytogenetic data on 22 new cases and review of the literature. Hum Genet 1986; 74:143-154.

39. Niikawa N, Ishikiriyama S, Takahashi S, Inagawa A, Tonoki H, Ohta Y, Hase N, Kamei T, Kajii T: The Wiedemann-Beckwith syndrome; Pedigree studies on five families with evidence for autosomal dominant inheritance with variable expressivity. Am J Med Genet 1986; 24:41-55.

40. Koufos A, Grundy P, Morgan K, Aleck KA, Hadro T, Lampkin BC, Kalbakji A, Cavenee WK: Familial Wiedemann-Beckwith syn-

drome and a second Wilms tumor locus both map to 11p15.5. Am J Hum Genet 1989; 44:711-719.

41. Ping AJ, Reeve AE, Law DJ, Young MR, Boehnke M, Feinberg AP: Genetic linkage of Beckwith-Wiedemann syndrome to 11p15. Am J Human Genet 1989; 44:720-723.

42. Waziri M, Patil S, Hanson J, Bartley SA: Abnormality of chromosome 11 in patients with features of Beckwith-Wiedemann syndrome. J Pediatr 1983; 102:873-876.

43. Turleau C, De Grouchy J, Chavin-Colin F, Martelli H, Charlas R: Trisomy 11p15 and Beckwith-Wiedemann syndrome: A report of two cases. Hum Genet 1984; 67:219-221.

44. Journel A, Lucas I, Allaire C, Le Mee F, Defawe G, Lecornu M, Jouan G, Roussey M, Le Marec B: Trisomy 11p15 and Beckwith-Wiedemann syndrome. Annales Genetique 1985; 28:97-101.

45. Okano Y, Osasa Y, Yamamoto H, Hase Y, Tsuruhara T, Fujita H: An infant with Beckwith-Wiedemann syndrome and chromosomal duplication 11p13-pter: Correlation of symptoms between 11p trisomy and Beckwith-Wiedemann syndrome. Jpn J Hum Genet 1986; 31:365-72.

46. Wales JHK, Walker V, Moore IE, Clayton PT: Bronze baby syndrome, biliary hypoplasia, incomplete Beckwith-Wiedemann syndrome and partial trisomy. Europ J Pediatr 1986; 145:141-5.

47. Henry I, Jeanpierre M, Couillin P, Barichard F, Serre JL, Jpurnel H, Lamouroux A, Turleau C, De Grouchy J, Junien C: Molecular definition of the 11p15.5 region involved in Beckwith-Wiedemann syndrome and probably in predisposition to adrenocortical carcinoma. Hum Genet 1989; 81:273-277.

48. Brown KW, Williams JC, N.J. M, Mott MG: Genomic imprinting and the Beckwith-Wiedemann syndrome. Am J Hum Genet 1990; 46:1000-1001.

49. Tonoki H, Narahara N, Marsumoto J, Niikawa N: Regional mapping of the parathyroid hormone gene (PTH) by cytogenetic and molecular studies. Cytogenet Cell Genet 1991; 56:103-4.

50. Henry I, Bonaiti-Pellie C, Chehensse V, Beldjord C, Schwartz C, Utermann G, Junien C: Uniparental paternal disomy in a genetic cancer-predisposing syndrome. Nature 1991; 351:665-667.

51. Grundy P, Telzerow P, Paterson MC, Haber D, Berman B, Li F, Garber J: Chromosome 11 uniparental isodisomy predisposing to embryonal neoplasms. Lancet 1991; 338:1079-1080.

52. Coppes MJ, Campbell CE, Williams BRG: The role of *WT1* in Wilms tumorigenesis. FASEB J 1993; 7:886-895.

53. Schroeder WT, Chao L-Y, Dao DD, Strong LC, Pathak S, Riccardi V, Lewis WH, Saunders GF: Nonrandom loss of maternal chromosome 11 alleles in Wilms tumors. Am J Hum Genet 1987; 40:413-20.

54. Wilkins RJ: Genomic imprinting and carcinogenesis. Lancet 1988; 1:329-331.

55. Surani MA, Barton SC, Norris ML: Experimental reconstruction of mouse eggs and embryos: an analysis of mammalian development. Biol Reproduct 1987; 36:1-16.
56. Reik W: Genomic imprinting and genetic disorders in man. Trends in Genet 1989; 5:331-336.
57. Shire JGM: Unequal parental contributions: genomic imprinting in mammals. The New Biologist 1989; 2:115-20.
58. Hall JG: Genomic imprinting: review and relevance to human diseases. Am J Hum Genet 1990; 46:857-873.
59. Reik W, Surani MA: Genomic imprinting and embryonal tumours. Nature 1989; 338:112-113.
60. Sapienza C, Peterson AC, Rossant J, Balling R: Degree of methylation of transgenes is dependent on gamete of origin. Nature 1987; 328:251-4.
61. Grundy P, Koufos A, Morgan K, Li FP, Meadows AT, Cavenee WK: Familial predisposition to Wilms' tumour does not map to the short arm of chromosome 11. Nature 1988; 336:374-376.
62. Huff V, Compton DA, Chao LY, Strong LC, Geiser CF, Saunders GF: Lack of linkage of familial Wilms' tumour to chromosomal band 11p13. Nature 1988; 336:377-378.
63. Schwartz CE, Haber DA, Stanton VP, Strong LC, Skolnick MH, Housman DE: Familial predisposition to Wilms tumor does not segregate with the *WT1* gene. Genomics 1991; 10:927-30.
64. Pelletier J, Bruening W, Li FP, Haber DA, Glaser T, Housman DE: *WT1* mutations contribute to abnormal genital system development and hereditary Wilms' tumour. Nature 1991; 353:431-434.
65. Haber DA, Buckler AJ, Glaser T, Call KM, Pelletier J, Sohn RL, Douglass EC, Housman DE: An internal deletion within an 11p13 zinc finger gene contributes to the development of Wilms' tumor. Cell 1990; 61:1257-1269.

CHAPTER 4

CLONING AND CHARACTERIZATION OF THE *WT1* LOCUS

INTRODUCTION

As described in chapter 1, patients with sporadic Wilms tumor suffer from aniridia at a frequency that is significantly greater than that seen in the general population. Conversely, about 33% of patients with severe sporadic aniridia develop Wilms tumor. These patients also have increased frequencies of genitourinary abnormalities and mental retardation resulting in the WAGR syndrome.[1] When these patients were studied with high resolution chromosome banding techniques, consistent chromosomal deletions of band p13 of the short arm of one of the two chromosomes 11 were noted,[1,2] suggesting that this region might contain a gene involved in the development of Wilms tumor (see chapter 3). Further evidence for the involvement of this region in Wilms tumor was provided by the observation that several patients with normal constitutional karyotypes demonstrated tumor-cell-specific deletions of 11p13.[3] The WAGR region was proposed to contain a cluster of genes that contribute to the development of the kidney, iris, genitourinary tract and nervous system.

The involvement of chromosome 11 in Wilms tumor was further supported by reports of tumor-specific loss of heterozygosity (LOH) of polymorphic chromosome 11 DNA probes suggesting the location of a potential recessive tumor suppressor gene (see chapter 3).

Wilms Tumor: Clinical and Molecular Characterization, by Max J. Coppes, Christine E. Campbell, and Bryan R.G. Williams. © 1995 R.G. Landes Company.

MAPPING OF THE WAGR REGION

The nature of different deletions in chromosome 11 homologues from different WAGR patients and the mapping of hybrid DNA panels carrying various deleted chromosome 11 DNAs suggested the size of this region was anywhere from 1 to 3 x 10^6 base pairs (bp), clearly large enough to harbor many genes. The first useful marker (and initially a candidate gene for Wilms tumor) for the WAGR locus was the gene for erythrocyte catalase (*CAT*). Based on dosage analysis of enzymatic activity in samples from patients having deletions and duplications of this area, the *CAT* gene was assigned to band p13,[4] a location subsequently confirmed by the mapping of the cDNA encoding *CAT* using in situ hybridization of metaphase chromosomes.[5] Subsequently it was shown that the gene encoding the β-subunit of follicle stimulating hormone (*FSHβ*) was deleted in patients with the WAGR syndrome.[6] Using these markers to delimit the region and several large deleted chromosome 11s isolated in hybrids as well as two non-identical translocations within 11p13 from two families with hereditary aniridia,[7] the order of the WAGR complex was established with respect to *CAT* and *FSHβ*. A cell surface antigen encoded by the gene *MIC1* was identified as the only gene lying within the WAGR locus and the relative order was suggested as: ...centromere...*CAT*...*MIC1*...*WT*...*AN2*...*FSHβ*[6,7] (Fig. 4.1).

A large number of additional DNA probes mapping to this region were identified through random screening methods using enrichment for chromosome 11 specific sequences and mapping these onto the different hybrid panels[8-12] allowing detailed 11p deletion maps to be established.

A more precise definition of the locus was provided by the isolation of a random DNA fragment, 2.3 (locus D11S87), which mapped between a translocation breakpoint associated with familial aniridia and another translocation breakpoint associated with childhood T-cell leukemia. The D11S87 locus was found to be homozygously deleted in a single case of sporadic Wilms tumor (WiT-13) identified at The Hospital for Sick Children in Toronto.[13] A cell line was developed from this tumor enabling the isolation of the maternal and paternal chromosomes in rodent cell hybrids. The probe D11S87 and the cell line WiT-13 provided a means of localizing the Wilms tumor locus on chromosome 11p13 and eventually led to the identification and cloning of candidate Wilms tumor genes independently by three groups.[14-16]

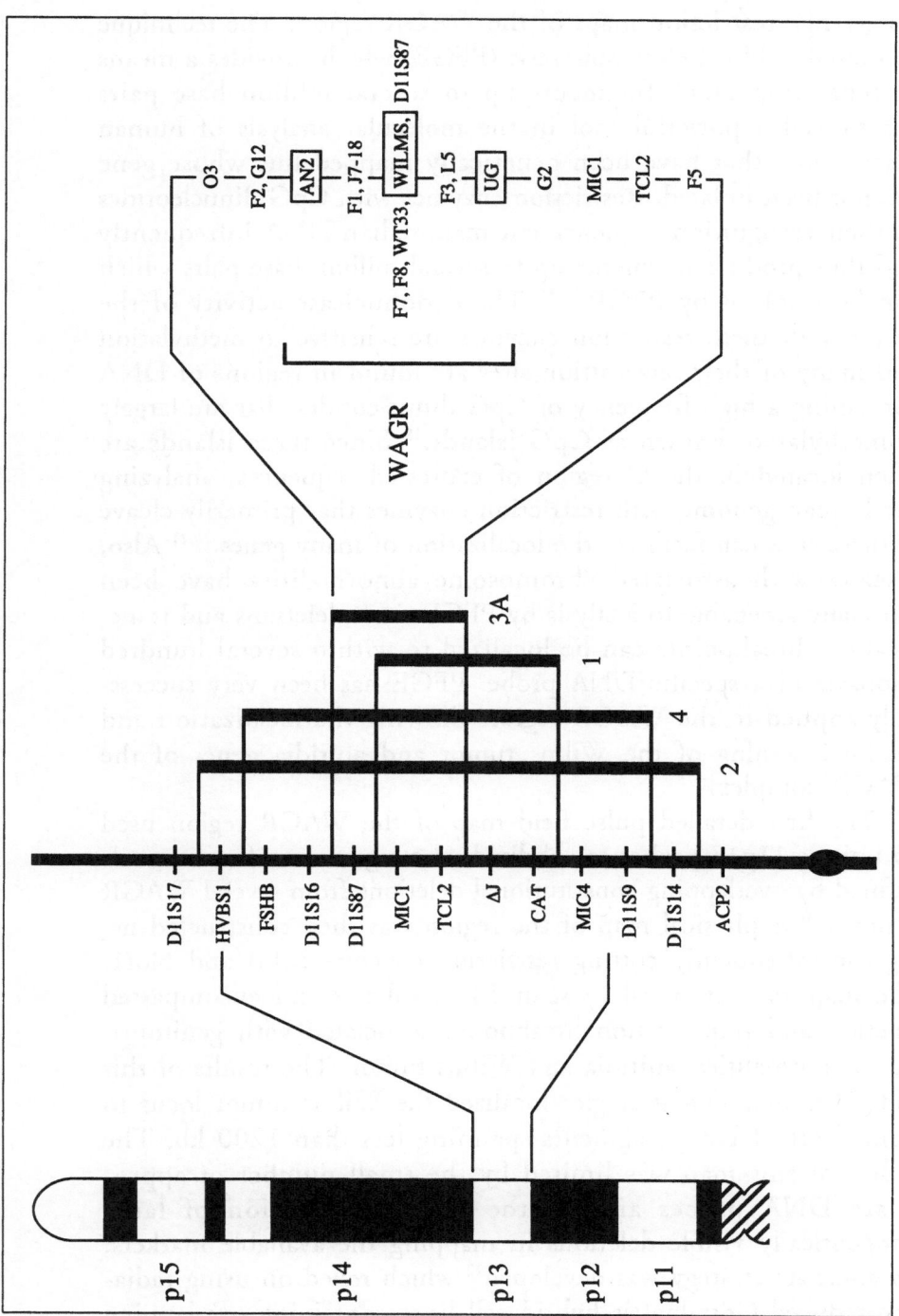

Fig. 4.1. Characterization of the WT1 locus using radiation-reduced hybrids derived from chromosome 11p13. The hybrids, depicted as vertical bars, were selected on the basis of retention of the MIC1 surface antigen and presence or absence of DNA markers from band p13. AN2 (aniridia gene, PAX6) UG (urogenital defects) and TCL2 (T-cell leukemia) are defined by constitutional translocations or breakpoints (TCL2) from individual patients (see ref. 14 and references therein for details).

The cloning of *WT1* was greatly aided by the construction of long-range restriction maps of the WAGR region. The technique of pulsed field gel electrophoresis (PFGE) which provides a means of separating DNA fragments up to several million base pairs has proved a powerful tool in the molecular analysis of human disease loci that have been genetically mapped but whose gene has not been isolated. Restriction enzymes with CpG dinucleotides in their recognition sequence cut mammalian DNA infrequently and thus produce fragments up to several million base pairs which can be resolved by PFGE.[17,18] The endonuclease activity of the majority of these restriction enzymes are sensitive to methylation and many of their recognition sites are found in regions of DNA containing a high frequency of CpG dinucleotides that are largely unmethylated, known as CpG islands.[19] Since these islands are often located in the 5' region of expressed sequences, analyzing the human genome with restriction enzymes that primarily cleave at these sites can facilitate the localization of many genes.[20,21] Also, diseases with associated chromosome abnormalities have been especially amenable to analysis by PFGE since deletions and trans-locations breakpoints can be localized to within several hundred kilobases of a specific DNA probe. PFGE has been very success-fully applied to the WAGR region allowing the localization and eventual cloning of the Wilms tumor and aniridia genes of the WAGR complex.

The first detailed pulse field map of the WAGR region used 15 unique 11p13 probes to subdivide the region into five intervals defined by overlapping constitutional deletions from several WAGR patients.[10] A physical map of the region was then constructed us-ing the infrequently cutting restriction enzymes MluI and Not1. The map was estimated to span 13 megabases and encompassed deletion and translocation breakpoints associated with genitouri-nary abnormalities, aniridia and Wilms tumor. The results of this and other mapping strategies localized the Wilms tumor locus to a small set of NotI fragments spanning less than 1200 kb. The utility of this map was limited by the small number of appro-priate DNA probes and by the limited resolution of large cytogentically visible deletions in mapping the available markers. An alternate strategy was developed[22] which relied on using radia-tion-reduced Goss-Harris hybrid cell lines containing overlapping portions of the WAGR region on chromosome 11p13 as physical mapping agents. The chromosome 11 in these hybrids was derived from a human-hamster hybrid line J1-11 which contained only the short arm of chromosome 11.[23] The radiation-reduced lines were obtained by exposing J1-11 cells to high doses of γ-radiation and rescuing the fragmented chromosomes by cell fusion with hamster cells. Cells containing the WAGR region of chromosome 11p were selected by panning with a monoclonal antibody against the cell surface antigen MIC1 previously localized to the WAGR region. The extent of human chromosome 11 DNA content of the resultant hybrid cell lines was characterized by hybridization to a panel of single-copy markers that had been previously mapped on chromosome 11[24,25] (Fig. 4.1).

The pulse field mapping data identified two adjacent NotI restriction fragments of 350 and 500 kb which likely housed the *WT1* gene. A series of 11p13-specific DNA probes were generated from genomic libraries constructed using the PFGE-selected NotI-digested DNA isolated from the hybrid cell lines. In total, eight probes plus D11S87 detected the 500 kb Not fragment and four probes detected the 350 kb fragment. These probes were used to refine the position of the Wilms tumor locus on the basis of the small homozygous deletion of 11p13 in the genome of WiT-13. The region of the deletion was estimated to be less than 350 kb. In addition it was noted the deletion removed a CpG island between the 500 and 350 kb Not1 fragments suggesting the *WT1* gene might be anchored to this island. This delineation of the limits of the *WT1* locus set the stage for chromosome walking and jumping from probes adjacent to the region

CLONING OF THE *WT1* GENE

The *WT1* gene on chromosome 11p13 was cloned using three independent but complimentary approaches. Housman and colleagues,[14,22] using PFGE mapping information and the position of marker S1 (*D1187*) within the shortest region of overlap defined by the Wilms tumor WiT-13, isolated cosmid clones within the WAGR region. Three cosmids were identified as mapping closest to the region containing the *WT1* gene. Single copy sequences were derived from these cosmids and mapped by hybridization to somatic cell hybrid panels derived from patients with translocations and deletions defining specific intervals within the WAGR region. Two of the probes were deleted in three constitutional

WAGR deletions, one was deleted in hybrids containing WiT-13 DNA and thus mapped to the region already identified by S1 as containing the Wilms tumor gene. Fortuitously, one of these probes, J8-3p4, showed strong cross-species hybridization to hamster and mouse genomic sequences and also hybridized to RNA isolated from baboon kidney and spleen. When this probe was used to screen cDNA libraries derived from embryonic kidney, adult kidney and pre-B cells, several cDNAs were isolated the longest of which, WT33, was 2313 bp. Nucleotide sequence analysis of this cDNA revealed a large continuous open reading frame which included a proline/glutamine-rich N-terminal domain and four contiguous zinc finger domains. These features are characteristic of a number of transcription factors including members of the early growth response (EGR) genes involved in pathways controlling cell proliferation. Preliminary characterization of the *WT1* gene indicated it spanned greater than 40 kb but lay within the 325 kb Not1 fragment with the 5' end of the gene mapping close to a CpG island marking the boundary between the 350 kb Not1 fragment and the more centromeric 500 kb Not1 fragment identified as harboring the S1 sequence.

In the same year, a combined approach of mapping CpG islands by PFGE and subsequent cloning by consecutive jumps from one island to another using rare cutting restriction-enzyme jumping libraries lead to the independent cloning of *WT1* by a second group of researchers headed by Bruns.[15] Their strategy relied on the observation that molecular probes for island associated genes should identify a significant number of expressed sequences. A random probe was chosen located close to the WAGR region and near two CpG islands and used for chromosome walking to isolate a new probe that contained one of the CpG islands. This island probe was then used to screen a BssHII-Eco RI jumping library resulting in the isolation of jumps in both directions (Fig. 4.2). Directionality of the jumps was established by mapping the new end fragments on somatic hybrid panels and by comparing the PFGE pattern with that of the starting clone. New jump fragments were used to isolate longer phage clones suitable for consecutive jumps. In this way, four neighboring CpG islands, all within 650 kilobases, were isolated from two consecutive bi-directional jumps in rare-cutting restriction enzyme jumping libraries. Several genomic fragments on either side of the CpG islands were assayed

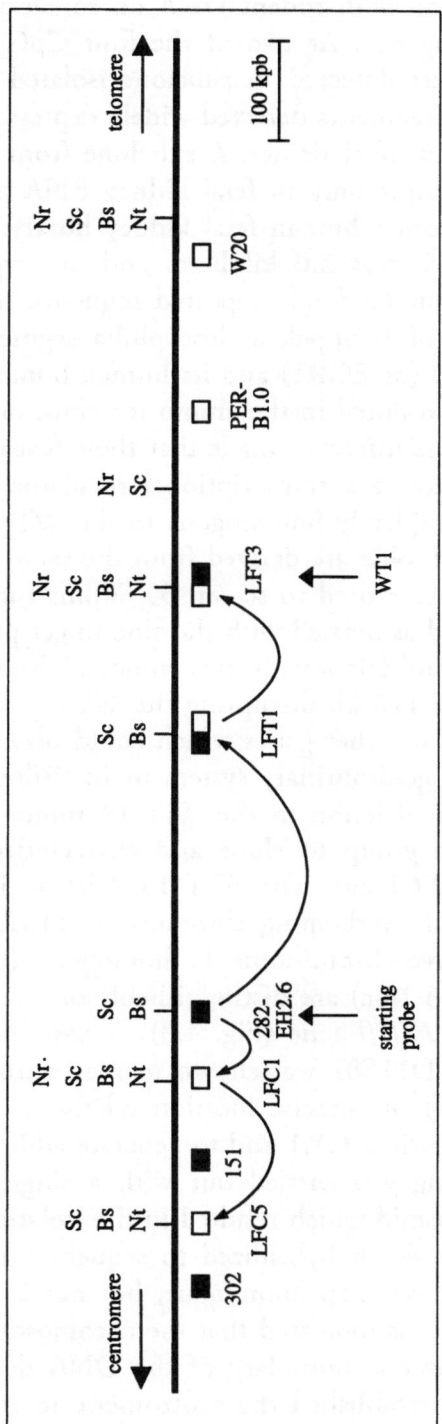

Fig. 4.2. Cloning of the WT1 gene by CpG island jumping. The solid line represents the physical map established by pulse field gel electrophoresis. The starting probe 282-EH2.6 was used to isolate four directional jumps. 302, 151, PER-B1.0 and W20 are random probes. The black boxes indicate conservation in rodent DNA. Adapted from Gessler et al.[15]

for cross-hybridization with rodent DNA on somatic hybrid panels under high stringency. At two of the four CpG islands conserved fragments were detected. A subclone isolated from one of the island genomic fragments detected widely expressed transcripts in RNA isolated from fetal tissues. A subclone from the other island detected transcripts only in fetal kidney RNA and was used to isolate cDNAs from a human fetal kidney library. The longest clone isolated, LK15, was 3.0 kilobases and on sequencing was found to contain four tandemly repeated sequence motifs related to the zinc fingers of Kruppel, a drosophilia segmentation gene and murine Krox-20 (or EGR1) and its human homolog. Proline-rich regions were also noted in the amino terminus of the putative coding region and the inference made that these features suggested that the cDNA encoded a transcriptional regulator. The LK 15 cDNA is almost completely homologous to the WT33 cDNA indicating that both cDNAs are derived from the same gene. All the CpG island clones were used to screen 65 Wilms tumors and the clone from the island associated with the zinc finger protein (*WT1*) identified homozygous deletions in two tumors. The two deletions overlapped by about 170 kb disrupting the *WT1* locus but allowing for the presence of other genes which could play a part in the development of the genitourinary system or in Wilms tumor.

The homozygous deletion in the WiT-13 tumor was also exploited by our own group to clone and characterize the cDNA mapping to the *WT1* locus. The WiT-13 deletion is defined by two independent but overlapping chromosome 11p13 deletions.[13] Each of the derivative chromosome 11 homolgues (termed WiT-13 Mac and WiT-13 Mic) are distinguishable on the basis of loss or retention of the *FSHβ* gene (Fig. 4.3). A cosmid clone, C1.1 which encompasses D11S87 was shown to map within the WiT-13 deletion, although its precise location relative to the deletion was not known. To orient C1.1 and to generate additional probes, chromosome jumping was carried out with a single copy probe isolated from this cosmid which resulted in the isolation of a single clone (J1, Fig. 4.4) which hybridized to sequences retained only in the WiT-13 Mac del 11p homologue, but not in the Mic del 11p. These observations indicated that the chromosome jump had traversed the centromeric boundary of the DNA deletion in the WiT-13 tumor and established the centromeric to telemeric map order of probes within the deletion and provided directionality to

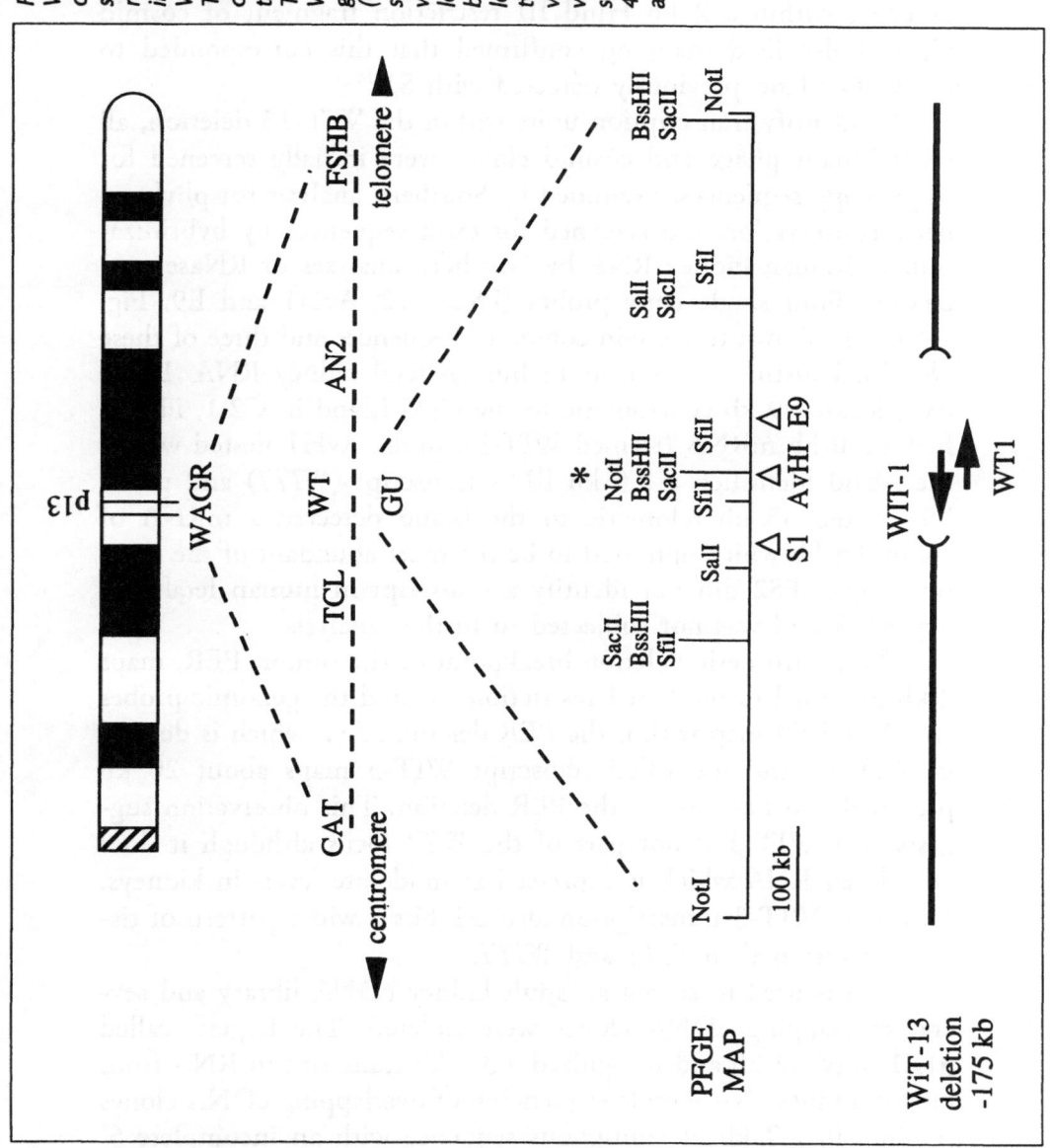

Fig. 4.3. The WT1 locus and WiT-13 deletion. The location of the WT1 and WIT1 genes are shown in relation to the homozygous deletion boundaries in the sporadic Wilms tumor, WiT-13 and the WAGR interval. The map order of the erythrocyte (CAT) catalase gene, the translocation associated with a T-cell leukemia (TCL), sporadic Wilms tumor (WT) deletions and genitourinary abnormalities (GU) and familial aniridia are shown. Pulse field mapping within the homozygously deleted region defined a minimal boundary for the Wilms tumor locus. The open arrows indicate two conserved probes in the vicinity of a CpG island (*) which were isolated by the chromosome walking detailed in Figure 4.4 and used to isolate the WT1 and WIT1 genes.

subsequent chromosome walking experiments. Bi-directional chromosome walking from S1 at D11S87 resulted in the cloning of contiguous sequences which spanned the WiT-13 deletion. A total of 13 phage and cosmid clones encompassing approximately 145 kb of DNA and the proximal WiT-13 deletion breakpoint were isolated and mapped. Eleven phage and cosmid clones spanning a contiguous DNA region of 130 kb were mapped to the WiT-13 delteion and a cluster of rare restriction cutting enzyme sites were detected within a 2 kb Hind III restriction fragment of cosmid C2.1. Pulse field mapping confirmed that this corresponded to the CpG island previously detected with S1.[16]

To identify transcription units within the WiT-13 deletion, all recombinant phage and cosmid clones were initially screened for single copy sequences, examined by Southern analysis for phylogenetic conservation and screened for exon sequences by hybridization to human kidney RNA by Northern analyses or RNase protection. Four single copy probes (PS2, Av2, AvH1 and E9, Fig. 4.4.) were shown to contain conserved sequences and three of these identified distinct transcripts in human fetal kidney RNA. Probe Av2, located 9 kb centromeric to the CpG island in C2.1, identified a 2.0 kb mRNA (termed WIT-3), probe AvH1 nested within the island identified a 2.5 kb RNA transcript (*WIT1*) and probe E9 located 35 kb telomeric to the island detected a mRNA of about 3.5 kb which appeared to be the most abundant of the three transcripts. PS2 did not identify a transcript in human fetal kidney RNA and was not subjected to further analysis.

The centromeric deletion breakpoint of the tumor, PER, maps 2 kb proximal to the Not I restriction site and the genomic probes AvH1 and E9 map within the PER deletion. Av2 which is deleted in WiT-13 and identified transcript WIT-3 maps about 20 kb proximal and lies outside the PER deletion. This observation suggests that WIT-3 is not part of the *WT1* locus although it does encode an RNA which is expressed at moderate levels in kidneys. However, WIT-3 transcription also exhibits a wider pattern of tissue expression than *WT1* and *WIT1*.

E9 was used to screen an adult kidney cDNA library and several overlapping cDNA clones were isolated. The largest, called 31E1, was 2.2 kb and recognized a 3.5 kb transcript in RNA from human kidney. Nucleotide sequencing of overlapping cDNA clones resulted in 2.7 kb of contiguous sequence with an incomplete 5'

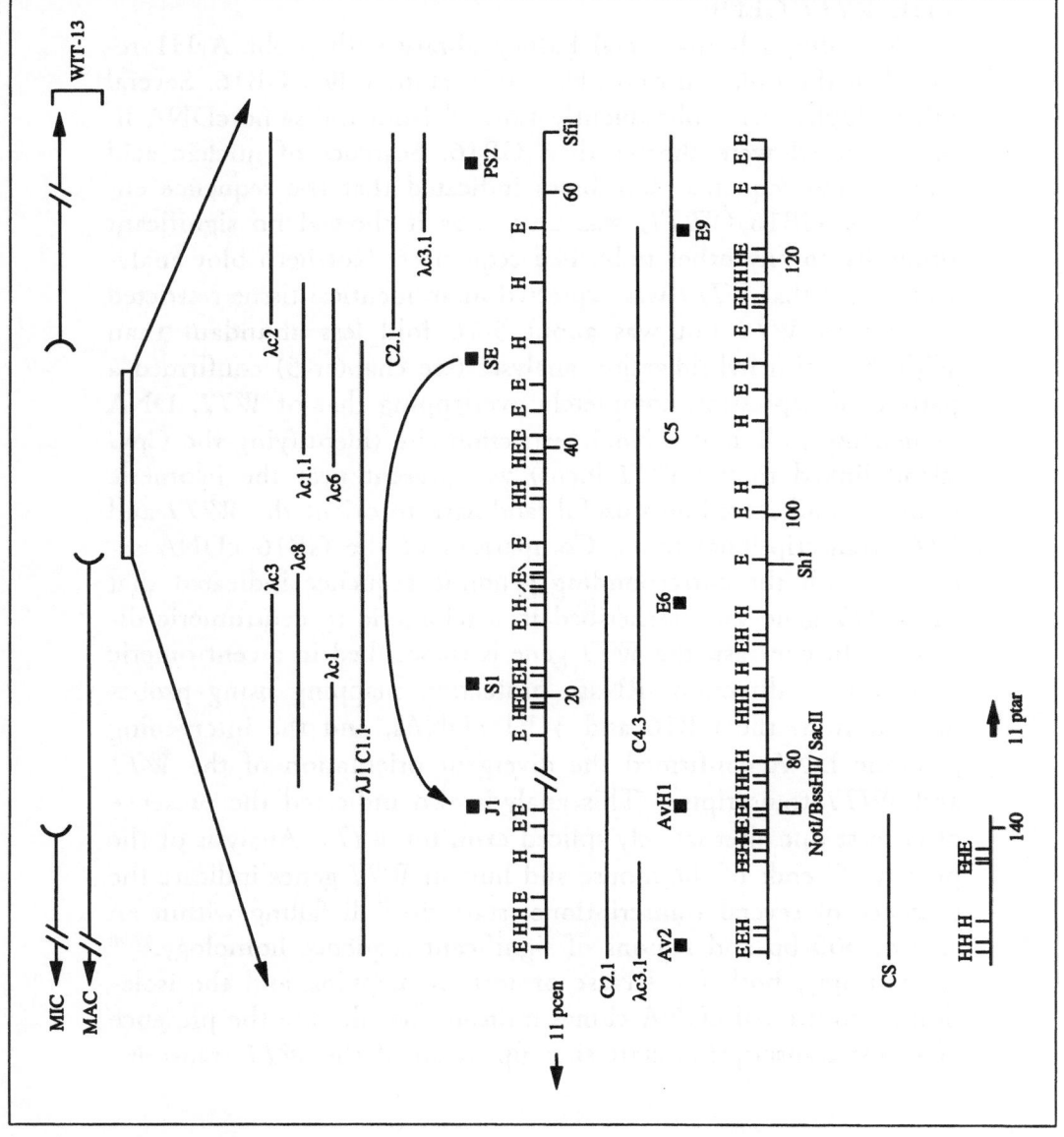

Fig. 4.4. Characterization of the WiT-13 deletion by chromosome walking. The top interrupted lines are a schematic representation of the maternal (MIC for micro deletion) and paternal (MAC for macro deletion) deleted chromosomes isolated from tumor WiT-13 and passaged in rodent hybrid cell lines. The region of homozygous deletion (rectangle) is expanded to show a detailed restriction endonuclease map of DNA cloned from this region and represented as cosmid (e.g., C1.1) and λ phage (e.g., λc1) clones. The restriction map of EcoRI (E) and HindIII (H) sites is shown from the left centromeric (11pcen) to the right telomeric (11pter) end. The distance in kilobase pairs is shown under the restriction enzyme sites. The CpG island within the WiT-13 deletion is shown as a open box with the cluster of rare restriction sites shown below. Sfi sites detected by PFGE and by restriction mapping of individual clones are also shown. The dark boxes show the position the unique copy probes S1, PS2, AV2, AVH1, E6 and E9. The chromosome jump which established directionality of the walk is shown by a curved arrow. The slashed line indicates sequences which were unstable when propagated as λ or cosmid clones. (Further details can be found in refs. 16 and 26).

end and a polyadenylated 3' terminus. 31E1 is also derived from
the *WT1* gene and 362 bp longer than WT33[14] and 272 bp shorter
than LK15.[15] Both 31E1 and LK15 contain two stretches of 51
and 9 nucleotides which are absent in WT33 and subsequently
shown to result from differential splicing of alternate exons (chapter 6). The longest open reading frame of 311E1 initiates with an
ATG codon at position 107. However it should be noted that this
ATG is not a good fit with a Kozak consensus, suggesting the
possibility of alternate transitional start sites.

THE *WIT1* GENE

Screening a human fetal kidney library with probe AvH1 resulted in the isolation of a 2kb cDNA clone called GB16. Several
other cDNA were subsequently isolated from the same cDNA library but all were shorter than GB16. Searches of nucleic acid
and protein sequence data bases indicated that the sequence encoded by GB16 (*WIT1*) was unique as it showed no significant
similarity to any other published sequences. Northern blot analysis revealed that *WIT1* was expressed in an identical tissue restricted
manner to *WT1* but was about 5-10 fold less abundant than
WT1.[26] In situ hybridization analyses (see chapter 5) confirmed a
pattern of expression completely overlapping that of *WT1*. DNA
sequencing indicated a Not1 restriction site (identifying the CpG
island linked to the *WT1* locus) was present near the telomeric
terminus and served as a useful landmark to orient the *WIT1* and
WT1 transcriptional units. Comparison of the GB16 cDNA sequence with the corresponding genomic sequence indicated that
the *WIT1* gene was transcribed in a telomeric to centromeric direction. In contrast, the *WT1* gene is transcribed in a centromeric
to telomeric direction. RNase protection mapping using probes
derived from the GB16 and 31E1 cDNAs, and the intervening
genomic DNA confirmed the divergent orientation of the *WT1*
and *WIT1* transcripts.[27] This analysis also indicated the presence
of at least one alternatively spliced exon for *WIT1*. Analysis of the
putative 5' ends of the mouse and human *WT1* genes indicate the
presence of several transcriptional start sites all falling within an
area of 300 bp and regions of significant sequence homology.[27,28]
Interestingly, both the RNase protection mapping and the isolation of additional cDNA clones indicate that despite the presence
of major transcription start sites upstream of the *WT1* transcrip-

tion initiation region, some *WIT1* transcripts include antisense sequences of the first exon of *WT1*. This is also a feature of the mouse *Wt1* locus (Bryan R.G. Williams, unpublished observations) and suggests that *WIT1* may play a role in the transcriptional control of the *WT1* gene.

The function of *WIT1* remains to be elucidated. The cDNA encodes multiple small open reading frames, the largest of which is not preceded by a Kozack consensus translation initiation signal. Moreover, translation of in vitro transcribed RNA derived from GB16 in either reticulocyte or wheat germ lysates does not yield a product. *WIT1* RNA was initially thought to be polyadenylated, but all cDNA characterized to date appear to terminate in a poly A tract in the genome. It remains possible that the *WIT1* gene product may function as an RNA. There is a mouse equivalent of *WIT1* and bi-directional transcription through the first exon of mouse *Wt1*. However there is little sequence homology between the human and mouse loci 5' of some shared upstream elements. This feature is also characteristic of the *H19* gene which may be translated in a very restricted developmental window but is thought to function as an RNA in a tumor suppressor assay.[29,30] It remains possible that the *WIT1* transcript is not functional but simply arises from cryptic promoter activation as a result of changes in chromatin structure because of cis-regulation of the adjoining *WT1* gene. The conservation of the transcript in the mouse, the complex splicing pattern and discordant expression of *WT1* and *WIT1* in some Wilms tumors makes this unlikely.[27] An alternative explanation that *WIT1* transcription may facilitate *WT1* transcription remains possible but has to be reconciled with the discordant pattern of expression seen in some tumors.[31] In the absence of a protein and with no functional assay for the RNA, any role for *WIT1* in Wilms tumorigenesis remains to be established. Wilms tumors which express no detectable *WIT1* RNA have been analyzed using a PCR based assay designed to detect small insertions or deletions within the *WIT1* sequence spanning the *WT1* 5' untranslated region and the *WIT1-WT1* transcriptional start sites but no alterations were detected. Clearly this has to be repeated using more sensitive detection methodologies. Ultimately however, the deletion of the mouse equivalent of *WIT1* using gene targeting strategies may be required to clearly establish its function in nephrogenesis and by implication the development of Wilms tumor.

PROMOTER REGION OF THE *WT1* LOCUS

WT1 transcription start sites cluster within a 300 bp genomic region that exhibits a high degree of sequence homology between human and mouse. The use of chimeric reporter constructs encompassing this region has identified basal promoter activity when assayed in the context of a strong enhancer.[27,32] With the exception of a possible enhancer element 3' of the *WT1* gene which may function specifically in cells of erythroid lineages,[33] no elements capable of conferring kidney specific expression have been identified. Multiple elements capable of interaction with nuclear proteins from WT1 expressing tissues have been defined by DNAse I protection assays but thus far the footprinted regions are indistinguishable between WT1 expressing and non-expressing tissues. Interestingly, WT1 itself binds to elements in its own promoter and may be autoregulatory.[32] Different consensus promoter elements including binding sites for the transcription factors Sp1, EGR-1 consensus motifs, an MLTF consensus sequence and SV40 enhancer core are all clustered in the basal promoter region. Since WT1 proteins bind different variations of these elements in vitro, and can be shown to footprint a region of the promoter containing the EGR-1 site, a functional role for these sites in *WT1* gene transcription seems likely. The two major human and murine *WT1* start sites can be aligned within regions of extensive sequence conservation. A primary *WT1* start site maps within a 100 bp pyrimidine-rich sequence characteristic of the nuclease sensitive regions found in many eukaryotic gene promoters. However, only weak transcriptional activity has been demonstrated using various promoter constructs in transfection assays suggesting that *WT1* is likely regulated by distal controlling elements. Alternatively, the constructs analyzed thus far may have to be tested in cell types which better reflect the differentiating cells expressing the endogenous *WT1* locus in vivo.

REFERENCES

1. Riccardi VM, Sujansky E, Smith AC, Francke U: Chromosomal imbalance in the aniridia-Wilms' tumor association: 11p interstitial deletion. Pediatrics 1978; 61:604-610.
2. Francke UL, Holmes LB, Atkins L, Riccardi VM: Aniridia-Wilms' tumor association: Evidence for specific deletion of 11p13. Cytogenet Cell Genet 1979; 24:185-192.

3. Kaneko Y, Egues MC, Rowley JD: Interstitial deletion of the short arm of chromosome 11 limited to Wilms tumor cells in a patient without aniridia. Cancer Res 1981; 41:4577-4578.

4. Junien C, Turleau C, G.M. L, Philip T, Said R, Despoisse S, Laurent C, Rethore MO, Kaplan JC, De Grouchy J: Catalase determination in various etiologic forms of Wilms' tumor and gonadoblastoma. Cancer Genet Cytogenet 1983; 10:51-57.

5. Schroeder WT, Chao L-Y, Dao DD, Strong LC, Pathak S, Riccardi V, Lewis WH, Saunders GF: Nonrandom loss of maternal chromosome 11 alleles in Wilms tumors. Am J Human Genet 1987; 40:413-20.

6. Glaser T, Lewis WH, Bruns GAP, Waltkins PC, Rogler CE, Shows TB, Powers VE, Willard HF, Goguen JM, Simola KO, Housman DE: The β subunit of follicle-stimulating hormone is deleted in patients with aniridia and Wilms' tumour, allowing a further definition of the WAGR locus. Nature 1986; 321:882-887.

7. Simola KO, Knuutila S, Kaitila I, Pirkola A, Pohja P: Familial aniridia and translocation t(4;1)(q22-p13) without Wilms tumor. Hum Genet 1983; 63:158-161.

8. Porteous DJ, Bickmore W, Christie S, Boyd PA, Cranston G, Fletcher JM, Gosden JR, Rout D, Seawright A, Simola KOJ, Van Heyningen V, Hastie ND: HRAS1-selected chromosome transfer generates markers that colocalize aniridia- and genitourinary dysplasia-associated translocation breakpoints and the Wilms tumor gene within band 11p13. Proc Natl Acad Sci USA 1987; 84:5355-5359.

9. Bickmore W, Christie S, Van Heyningen V, Hastie ND, Porteous DJ: Hitch-hicking from HRAS to the WAGR locus with CMGT markers. Nucl Acid Res 1988; 16:51-60.

10. Compton DA, Weil MM, Jones C, Riccardi VM, Strong LC, Saunders GF: Long range physical map of the Wilms' tumor-aniridia region on human chromosome 11. Cell 1988; 55:827-836.

11. Davis LM, Everest A, Simola OJ, Shows TB: Long-range restriction map around the 11p13 aniridia locus. Somatic Cell Mol Genet 15:605-615, 1989.

12. Gessler M, Bruns GAP: A physical map around the WAGR complex on the short asm of chromosome 11. Genomics 1989; 5:43-55.

13. Lewis WH, Yeger H, Bonetta L, Chan HLS, Kang J, Junien C, Cowell J, Jones C, Dafoe LA: Homozygous deletion of a DNA marker from chromosome 11p13 in sporadic Wilms tumor. Genomics 1988; 3:25-31.

14. Call KM, Glaser T, Ito CY, Buckler AJ, Pelletier J, Haber DA, Rose EA, Kral A, Yeger H, Lewis WH, Jones C, Housman DE: Isolation and characterization of a zinc finger polypeptide gene at the human chromosome 11 Wilms' tumor locus. Cell 1990; 60:509-520.

15. Gessler M, Poustka A, Cavenee W, Neve RL, Orkin SH, Bruns GA: Homozygous deletion in Wilms tumours of a zinc-finger gene identified by chromosome jumping. Nature 1990; 343:774-778.

16. Bonetta L, Kuehn SE, Huang A, Law DJ, Kalikin LM, Koi M, Reeve AE, Brownstein BH, Yeger H, Williams BRG, Feinberg AP: Wilms tumor locus on 11p13 defined by multiple CpG island-associated transcripts. Science 1990; 250:994-997.

17. Carle GF, Olsen MV: Separation of chromosomal DNA from yeast by orthogonal-field-gel electrophoresis. Nucl Acids Res 1984; 12:5947-5964.

18. Schwartz DC, Cantor C: Separation of yeats chromosome-sized DNAs by pulse field gel electrophoresis. Cell 1984; 37:67-75.

19. Brown WR, Bird AP: Long-range restriction site mapping of mammalian genomic DNA. Nature 1986; 322:477-481.

20. Bird AP: CpG-rich islands and the function of DNA methylation. Nature 1986; 321:209-213.

21. Lindsay S, Bird AP: Use of restriction enzymes to detect potential gene sequences in mammalian DNA. Nature 1987; 327:336-338.

22. Rose EA, Glaser T, Jones C, Smith CL, Lewis WH, Call KM, Minden M, Champagne E, Bonetta L, Yeger H, Housman DE: Complete physical map of the WAGR region of 11p13 localizes a candidate Wilms' tumor gene. Cell 1990; 60:495-508.

23. Jones C, Kao TT: Regional mapping of the gene for human lysosomal acid phosphatase using hybrid clones containing segments of human chromosome 11. Hum Genet 1978; 45:1-10.

24. Glaser T, Housman D, Lewis WH, Gerhard D, Jones C: A fine-structure deletion map of human chromosome 11p: analysis of J1 series hybrids. Somat Cell Mol Genet 1989; 15:477-501.

25. Glaser T, Rose E, Morse H, Housman D, Jones C: A panel of irradiation-reduced hybrids selectively retaining human chromosome 11p13: their structure and use to purify the WAGR gene complex. Genomics 1990; 6:48-64.

26. Huang A, Campbell CE, Bonetta L, McAndrews -Hill M, Chilton-MacNeill S, Coppes MJ, Law DJ, Feinberg AP, Yeger H, Williams BRG: Tissue, developmental, and tumor-specific expression of divergent transcripts in Wilms tumor. Science 1990; 250:991-994.

27. Campbell CE, Huang A, Gurney AL, Kessler PM, Hewitt JA, Williams BRG: Antisense transcripts and protein binding motifs within the Wilms tumour (*WT1*) locus. Oncogene 1994; 9:583-595.

28. Pelletier J, Schalling M, Buckler AJ, Rogers A, Haber DA, Housman D: Expression of the Wilms' tumor gene *WT1* in the murine urogenital system. Genes Dev 1991; 5:1345-1356.

29. Hao Y, Crenshaw T, Moulton T, Newcomb E, Tycko B: Tumour-suppressor activity of *H19* RNA. Nature 1993; 365:764-767.

30. Leibovitch MP, Nguyen VC, Gross MS, Solhonne B, Leibovitch SA, Bernheim A: The human ASM (Adult Skeletal Muscle) gene: expression and chromosomal assignment to 11p15. B B Res Comm 1991; 180:1241-1250.

31. Yeger H, Cullinane C, Flenniken A, Chilton-MacNeill S, Campbell C, Huang A, Bonetta L, Coppes MJ, Thorner P, Williams BRG: Coordinate expression of Wilms tumor genes correlates with Wilms tumor phenotypes. Cell Growth Differentiation 1992; 3:855-864.
32. Rauscher III FJ: The *WT1* Wilms tumor gene product: A developmentally regulated transcription factor in the kidney that functions as a tumor suppressor. FASEB 1993; J 7:896-903.
33. Fraizier GC, Wu Y-J, Hewitt SM, Maity T, Ton CCT, Huff V, Saunders GF: Transcriptional regulation of the human Wilms tumor gene (*WT1*). J Biol Chem 1994; 269:8892-8900.

CHAPTER 5

DEVELOPMENTAL AND TISSUE-SPECIFIC EXPRESSION PATTERNS OF THE WILMS TUMOR SUPPRESSOR GENE *WT1*

INTRODUCTION

The association of urogenital abnormalities with Wilms tumor in the WAGR syndrome suggested a possible role for *WT1* in normal urogenital development. As discussed in chapter 1, patients with Wilms tumor and genitourinary abnormalities present at an early age, as do those with bilateral Wilms tumor and those with associated ILNRs. This observation suggests an inherited genetic defect in these patients. The isolation of the *WT1* gene has provided an opportunity to test the prediction that the gene implicated in Wilms tumors originating from chromosome 11p13 genetic events, may be important in genitourinary development.

We now know that heterozygous germline mutations in *WT1* can give rise to a phenotype which includes nephropathy, urogenital abnormalities and Wilms tumor (Denys-Drash syndrome, DDS, see chapter 7), suggesting that the urogenital system is very sensitive to *WT1* levels during development. Thus, aberrant *WT1* expression can indeed result in developmental abnormalities affecting the urogenital system.

Initial RNA blot analyses indicated higher expression of *WT1* in fetal than in adult kidney and a restricted tissue distribution[1,2] (see below). In situ analyses of *WT1* mRNA on human fetal material

Wilms Tumor: Clinical and Molecular Characterization, by Max J. Coppes, Christine E. Campbell, and Bryan R.G. Williams. © 1995 R.G. Landes Company.

confirmed the restricted tissue distribution and indicated strong expression in the mesonephric and metanephric kidney and in the developing gonad.

The temporal and spatial distribution of *WT1* expression during embryogenesis, has been examined in more detail using in situ mRNA hybridization and immunohistochemistry in murine embryos during the period prior to and throughout active organogenesis. This analysis confirms that *WT1* mRNA levels correlate with the presence of specific histopathologic features of Wilms tumor which resemble early morphologic features of nephrogenesis.[1,3,4] The expression pattern of *WT1* in genitourinary development has been examined in the human, rat, and mouse,[5-9] and shows *WT1* gene expression is restricted to the developing genitourinary system, spleen, mesothelium, dorsal mesentery of the intestines, muscle and central nervous system. Thus *WT1* is tissue-restricted with differential expression occurring during certain stages of development.

WT1 mRNA EXPRESSION DURING EARLY EMBRYOGENESIS

In the developing mouse, the end of the blastocyst stage (and the beginning phase of elemental organogenesis) is marked by the formation of the trilaminar embryo and subsequent development of the neural tube, which occurs between embryonic day 7.5 (E7.5) and E9.5. At this point in time in murine embryogenesis, *WT1* mRNA expression is absent in the embryo; nor is expression detected either within the extraembryonic membranes or the trophoblastic cells.[10] However, high levels of *WT1* expression can be seen throughout the maternal endometrium (Figs. 5.1A and B).

The period in which the earliest mesodermal derivatives which will differentiate into mesothelium, the spleen, and the genitourinary systems appear, is also characterized by lack of *WT1* expression in the murine embryo.[11] During the process of gastrulation, when the bilaminar embryonic disc composed of endoderm and ectoderm is converted into a trilaminar embryonic disc by the addition of mesoderm,[10] no *WT1* expression is detected in the mesodermal, endodermal or ectodermal cells.[11] Furthermore, no *WT1* expression is seen (Figs. 5.1A and B) during the formation of the neural tube (E8.5 and E9.5). Subsequently, when the cells of the three germ layers divide, migrate and differentiate into the

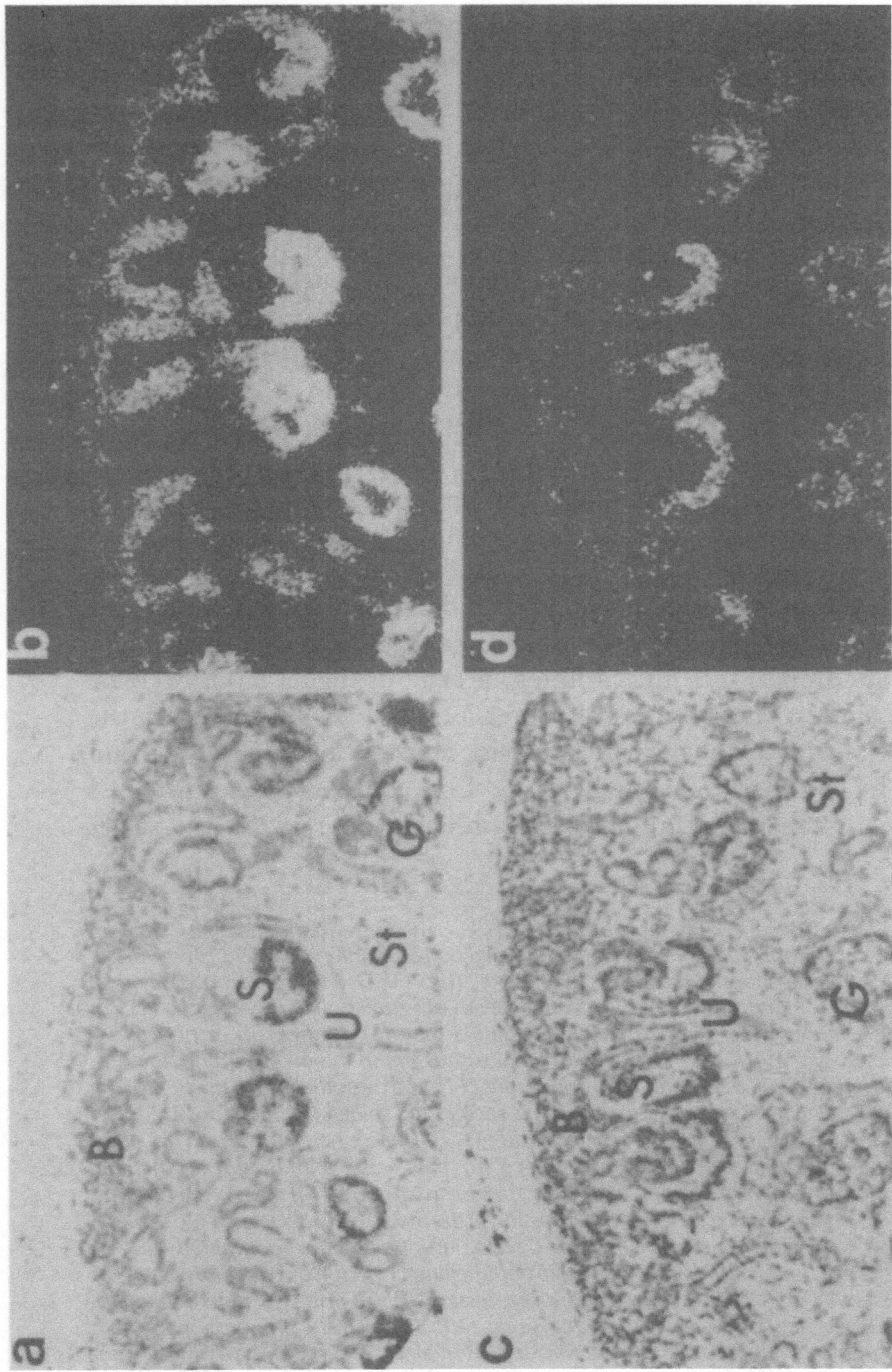

Fig. 5.1. Expression of WT1 and WIT1 in normal human fetal kidney. The blastema (B), S-tubules (S), and glomeruli (G) show expression of both WT1 and WIT1. The stroma (St) and ureteric bud (U) do not express WT1 or WIT1. The localization of WT1 (a,b) and WIT1 (c,d) was determined by in situ hybridization using ³H-labeled probes. Sections were photographed with bright-field illumination (left) to depict the morphology and with dark-field illumination (right) to show hybridization signals. Reprinted with permission from Yeger H et al. Coordinate expression of Wilms tumor genes correlates with Wilms tumor phenotypes. Cell Growth & Differentiation 1992; 3:855-864. Copyright © American Association for Cancer Research, Inc.

tissues and organs of the embryo as described below, again no expression of *WT1* gene is seen in these early blastic derivatives. The earliest expression of *WT1* is found restricted to the lateral lining of the intraembryonic intermediate mesoderm at E9 (13 somite stage).[8]

EXPRESSION OF *WT1* mRNA DURING ORGANOGENESIS

Following the stages of gastrulation and neurulation, the embryo enters the embryonic and fetal phase of organogenesis.[10] By E10.5 (equivalent to E27-33 in humans), rudimentary organogenesis has preceded in a cranio-caudal direction and *WT1* expression becomes clearly localized (Fig. 5.2).[11] Intense *WT1* expression is seen in the pleuropericardial (thoracic) cavity, both in the parietal (outer) and visceral mesothelial lining of the thymus, heart and lung. The intensity of *WT1* expression in the parietal and visceral mesothelial lining of all the organs within the peritoneal (abdominal) cavity is similar to that in the thoracic cavity. Because the dorsal mesentery of the abdominal organs is composed of two layers of peritoneal mesothelial lining, it exhibits higher levels of *WT1* expression.[11] The mesothelial expression of *WT1* within either the thoracic or abdominal cavities remains constant between E10.5 and E16.5. The mesothelial cells differ from cells of other epithelial surfaces in that they are derived from embryonic mesoderm rather

---

Fig. 5.2. Expression of WT1 in mouse embryos. A, C, E and G are Toluidene Blue O stained brightfield photomicrographs. B, D, F and H are corresponding darkfield photomicrographs. Sagittal sections of E8.5 (A, B: X 30), E10.5 (C: X 60, D: X 68) and E11.5 (E, F: X 60 and G, H: X 125) are shown. A, B show high levels of expression in the decidua (1) but not in the amnion (2), neuroepithelium of neural tube (3), somites (4) or pericardio-peritoneal cavity (5). C, D show high levels of expression in the mesonephric duct (9), urogenital ridge (10), degenerating pronephrons (11), and mesothelium of the peritoneal and thoracic cavity (18). Lower expression is seen in the spleen (7), midgut with dorsal mesentery (16) and mesentery of urogenital ridge (17). There is no expression in the other areas noted including the lumen of stomach (6), pancreatic primordium (8), hepatic primordium (liver, 12), first branchial arch (13), pericardial cavity (14) main bronchus with lung bud (15). E, F show high levels of expression in the metanephric blastema (20), spleen (7), mesentery of urogenital ridge (17) and developing infro-anterior abdominal wall (23), but not in the ureteric bud and surrounding epithelium (19), dorsum of embryo (21), or iliac vessels (22). G, H illustrate high levels of expression of WT1 in the germinal epithelium (24), and mesonephric vesicle with podocyte cap (25), but not in the primordial germ cells (26). Reprinted with permission from Rackley RR et al. Expression of the Wilms' tumor suppressor gene WT1 during mouse embryogenesis. Cell Growth & Differentiation 1993; 4:1023-1031. Copyright © American Association for Cancer Research, Inc.

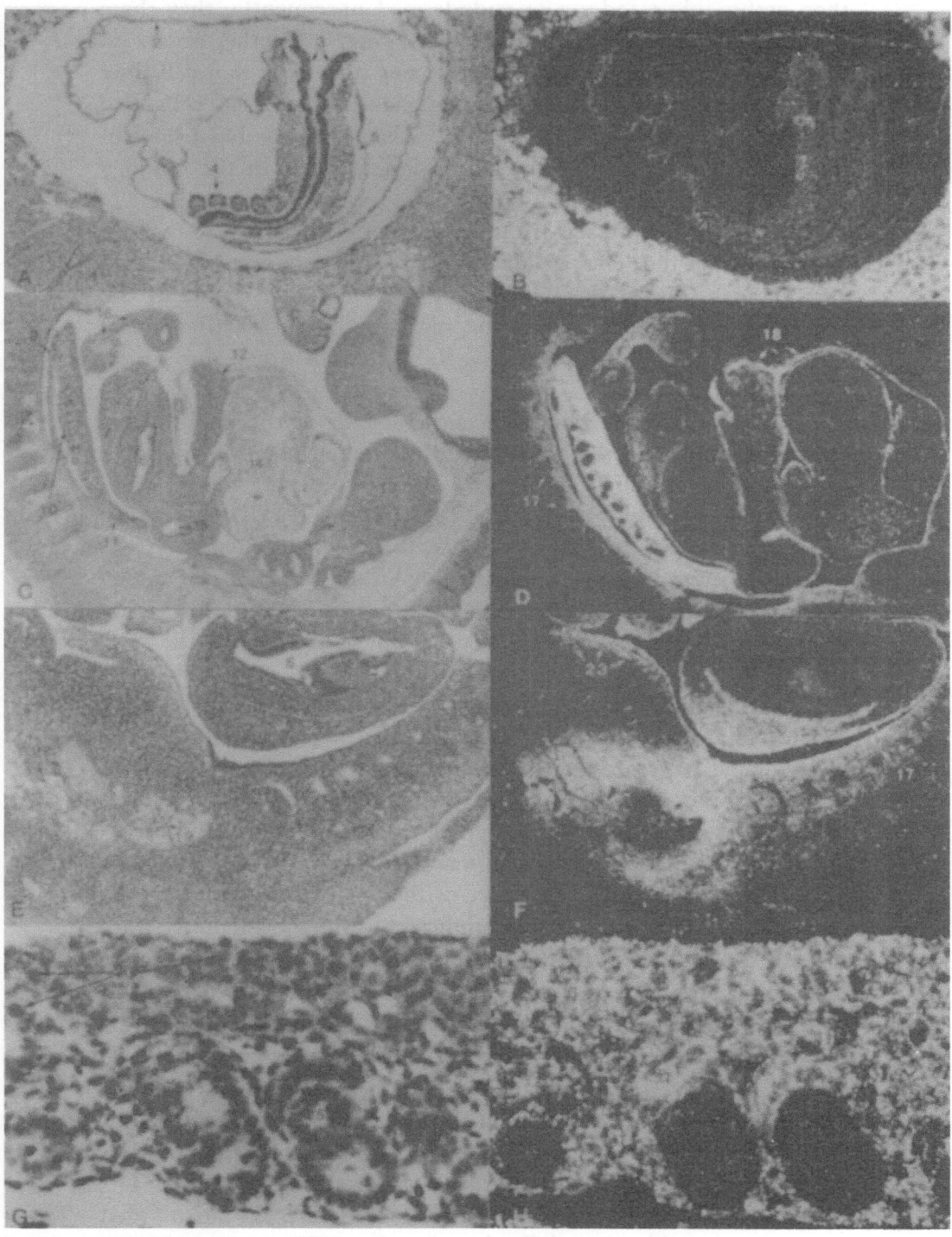

than embryonic ectoderm or endoderm. Consequently, they share a common embryonic origin with the kidney and other organs of the genitourinary tract. It is therefore not surprising that cell lines derived from both normal and malignant mesothelial cells also express high levels of *WT1* mRNA.[12] Also, evidence has been obtained supporting a role for inactivation of *WT1* in the etiology of certain mesotheliomas.[12]

WT1 is not expressed within organs of endodermal derivation which include the liver, gallbladder, stomach, pancreas, intestines and bladder (Fig. 5.2). Interestingly, although the cortex of the adrenal gland develops from the mesoderm, *WT1* expression is restricted to the outer mesothelial lining of this organ during development (E10.5-E16.5).[11]

WT1 is expressed along the entire length of the nephrogenic cord extending from the cranium to the urethral plate. While *WT1* expression occurs in the urogenital mesentery during the development of the pronephric and mesonephric structures (E10.5-E11.5), *WT1* is not expressed within the dorsal body wall when the rudimentary excretory organs undergo involution and replacement by the metanephric tissue (E12.5). *WT1* expression occurs in the developing abdominal wall musculature but is limited to the dorsal aspect of the anterior abdominal wall.

The bilateral nephrogenic cords produce longitudinal bulges referred to as urogenital ridges which are the origins of both nephric and gonadal structures.[10] All three different but temporal overlapping developmental organs of the urinary excretory system express *WT1*.[11] Within the genitourinary ridge, the pronephric and mesonephric structures surrounding the nephric duct show intense *WT1* expression by E10.5. Cellular caps of the mesonephric ducts which resemble the podocyte differentiation within the metanephric structures of the permanent kidney exhibit high *WT1* expression. Within the caudal aspect of the retroperitoneum, condensation of metanephric mesoderm around the ureteric bud signals the earliest formation of the permanent kidney. By E12.5, the pronephri and mesonephri have involuted and the metanephri begin their development and "ascent" to the cranial aspect of the retroperitoneum. Very early (E12.5) the ureteric bud expands within the tissue of the metanephric blastema to form the primitive renal pelvis. The branching ureteric buds form major calyces which are surrounded by metanephric blastema diffusely expressing *WT1*. Between E13.5

and E16.5, *WT1* expression parallels the centripetal differentiation of renal development. Low *WT1* expression occurs in the cortex of the kidney where the metanephric blastema resides. *WT1* expression increases as the metanephric blastema undergoes differentiation into renal vesicle and podocyte formation. *WT1* expression is restricted to the epithelial caps of mature glomeruli of well differentiated metanephrons. No *WT1* expression is found within the remaining structures of the nephron which include the proximal and distal convoluted tubules, and the loop of Henle.

Although the ureteric bud and metanephric blastema both arise from the intermediate mesoderm, no expression of *WT1* occurs in the epithelial lining of the collecting system and ureter which are derivatives of the ureteric bud. It is of interest that the differentiated epithelial cells of the pronephric, mesonephric and paramesonephric structures such as the mesonephron tubules, the common nephric duct, the efferent ductules of the testis, and the lining of the uterus and oviduct do not express *WT1* during development. The bladder and posterior urethra also do not express *WT1* within epithelial and supporting tissue structures.

Expression of the WT1 protein (detected by immunofluorescence staining) during renal development parallels *WT1* mRNA expression.[11] Consequently, the presence of the WT1 protein is also highly tissue-restricted and follows a specific expression pattern during renal development. Thus, WT1 protein is found associated with glomerular podocytes and their precursors derived from the metanephric blastema. Nuclear localization of WT1, shows the protein within the podocyte epithelium of the developing glomeruli, although polyclonal WT1 antibodies also detect some cytoplasmic staining. However, consistent with the results obtained by in situ hybridization using antisense RNA probes, immunofluorescent antibody detection of the WT1 protein is seen in the cytoplasm and nuclei of identical cell types. Interestingly, the WT1 protein is still detected in adult glomerular podocytes. It has been suggested that WT1 might have a function in maintaining the homeostasis of mature glomeruli.[13] If indeed this is the case, this could explain the development of the characteristic nephropathy which develops after the completion of nephrogenesis, seen in patients with Denys-Drash syndrome (DDS, see chapter 7). Possibly, the DDS-associated nephropathy results as a failure of WT1 to maintain normal podocyte function.

WT1 EXPRESSION IN SPLEEN
AND LYMPHOID DERIVATIVES

The spleen is a derivative of mesoderm which exhibits differential *WT1* expression during the earliest detectable stage of splenic development (E10.5, see Fig. 5.2) when the spleen and stomach share a common mesentery. As the spleen becomes more organized in its appearance and develops a separate blood supply, *WT1* expression increases, albeit localized to the capsule and epithelial supporting reticular tissue of the spleen; *WT1* expression is not detected in splenocytes.

While normal adult splenic B and T cells do not express *WT1*, a number of malignant hematopoietic cells of all lineages do contain elevated levels of *WT1* mRNA. These include acute lymphoblastic leukemia (ALL), acute myeloblastic leukemia (AML) and chronic myelogenous leukemia (CML) in blast crisis.[14] Because *WT1* expression seems to be limited to leukemia cells with associated immature hematopoietic precursors, it has been suggested that *WT1* expression may be involved in the early stages of hematological cell differentiation.[14] Recently, evaluation of *WT1* mRNA expression in patients with ALL, AML, CML, acute mixed lineage leukemia and non-Hodgkins lymphoma, has revealed that *WT1* expression might possibly be used as a prognostic factor in acute leukemia.[15] In addition, however, Inoue and colleagues demonstrated that *WT1* mRNA expression might also be used to detect minimal residual disease.[15] Mutation analysis indicated the absence of *WT1* mutations in all patients studied. Therefore, it seems likely that the *WT1* expression levels in these tumors reflect the presence of immature leukemic cells, possibly resistant to therapy.[15] The presence of WT1 protein has thus far not been demonstrated in leukemic cells. In addition, it remains to be seen whether manipulation of *WT1* expression in leukemic cell lines could alter their phenotypes. However, *WT1* mRNA can be down-regulated during the induction of differentiation of K562 cells along the erythroid or megakaryocytic lineages[16] or differentiation of HL60 cells along granulocytic or monocytic lineages.[17] These data are consistent with a role for *WT1* in maintaining these cells in the undifferentiated, proliferating state perhaps by repressing genes required for maturation. Again this observation still needs to be confirmed at the protein level. Similarly, experiments evaluating whether direct inhibition of *WT1* expression in undifferentiated cells induces a differentiated phenotype remain to be performed.

GONADAL EXPRESSION OF *WT1*

Murine gonadal development begins along the antero-medial aspect of the urogenital ridge.[18] During the early indifferent stage of gonadal development, intense *WT1* expression is seen in the developing mouse embryo at E10.5 within the proliferating coelomic epithelial cells and the underlying mesenchyme of the gonadal ridge.[11] Ensuing development of the gonad results in *WT1* expression being restricted to the supporting Sertoli (sustentacular) cells and tunica albuginea of the testes, and the granulosa cells and surface epithelium of the ovaries. The supporting tissue of the paramesonephric and mesonephric duct also shows high *WT1* expression throughout the embryonic period of E10.5 to E16.5 as demonstrated in Figure 5.2.[11]

As expected, immunofluorescent staining of the testes and uterus demonstrate the presence of the WT1 protein, paralleling *WT1* mRNA expression in these organs. The WT1 protein is also seen throughout the developing human ovary with the most pronounced expression in the epithelial layer surrounding the ovary.

WT1 EXPRESSION DURING DECIDUAL DIFFERENTIATION

As noted above, *WT1* is expressed in the maternal uterus. From studies in the rat, this appears to be mainly in the prepubertal uterine stromal cells and in decidual cells.[19] *WT1* mRNA is also found in uterine stromal fibroblasts during postnatal maturation of the uterus. However, its expression decreases with sexual maturity. Uterine levels remains low until the time of blastocyst implantation when the onset of decidualization induces *WT1* gene expression by stromal cells in a distinct spatio-temporal pattern. *WT1* expression then persists throughout the entire decidua at high levels throughout pregnancy. WT1 protein detected by immunocytochemistry is localized to the nuclei of the decidual cells. Although these data suggest a role for *WT1* in the differentiation of uterine stromal cells into decidual cells, the mechanism of action of the WT1 protein in this system remain to be determined. Although IGF2 or IGF2-receptor can be repressed by *WT1* in vitro, there appears to be no correlation in the expression of *WT1* and either of these genes in the differentiation of rat decidua.

In addition to *WT1* expression in the maternal uterus, there is also expression of *WT1* in the embryonic uterus as early as E13.5.[6,8,11] The highest intensity of uterine *WT1* expression appears around the endometrial cavity but uterine expression continues throughout gestation. While the body of the uterus and the uterine horn expresses *WT1*, there is no expression in the inner epithelial lining of these structures.[11]

WT1 EXPRESSION IN THE BRAIN

In the central nervous system there is low *WT1* expression within the ventral aspect of the spinal cord throughout its cranial and caudal extent.[11] This *WT1* expression is localized to the ependymal layer at E12.5 and E13.5. Immunocytochemistry shows WT1 immunoreactivity in the spinal cord in a location possibly representing ependymal cells suggesting a role for *WT1* in epithelial differentiation in the spinal cord. It should be noted however that in the early stage of neuronal development, no *WT1* expression occurs during neurotube formation.

In addition, *WT1* expression within derivatives of ectoderm suggests a possible role of the *WT1* gene in the development of the nervous system.[8,9] The localization of *WT1* within the ependymal layer of the spinal cord and in the fourth ventricle in areas with overlying ependymal cells (the area postrema and choroid plexus) supports this notion.[8,9] To date, localization studies have demonstrated area-specific expression but have not detailed the cell specific expression of *WT1* within the central nervous system. Expression of a tissue-restricted gene such as *WT1* in both mesodermal and ectodermal derived tissues seems odd but it could be that *WT1* expression in the germinal ependymal lining cells may be responsible for the induction of well-differentiated epithelium such as mature ependymal cells.

WT1 AND EARLY UROGENITAL DEVELOPMENT

The role of *WT1* in urogenital development has been directly addressed by generating mice with a targeted mutation in the *WT1* gene.[20] While animals carrying a heterozygous mutation developed normally, homozygotes exhibited embryonic lethality. The cause of death of these embryos was likely due to a major hemodynamic abnormality possibly because of abnormal heart development leading to right-sided congestive heart failure.[20] However the primary defect which contributes to this phenotype remains to be uncovered, especially because *WT1* is not expressed in the myocardium. Nevertheless, *WT1* expression has been reported in the pericardium, likely representing expression in the mesothelium. Since the mesothelium is derived from mesoderm, *WT1* possibly plays a role in the mesenchymal to epithelial transition and its absence results in abnormalities in all organs associated with this specialized tissue. This hypothesis is supported by the demonstration that the pleural cavity in homozygously mutated animals does not grow to an extent sufficient to allow normal lung development.

Development of the gonads is also severely affected in *WT1* mutant embryos, however migration of primordial germ cells to the urogenital ridge remains unaltered.[20] It appears that *WT1* is required for early commitment to and maintenance of gonadogenesis. Perhaps the most striking observation made in the *WT1* mutant mice is the arrest in kidney development following the establishment of metanephric blastema from intermediate mesoderm.[20] Although the metanephric blastema is present at E11, apoptosis is detected in a much larger fraction of cells than was seen in wild-type embryos, and by E12 no mesenchymal cells are apparent. Experiments performed with cultured rudiments from the mutant embryos showed that these were not stimulated to differentiate by spinal chord, a known powerful inducer of tubular induction,[20] suggesting that *WT1* plays an essential role in the induction process during nephrogenesis. While the molecular defects resulting from the ablation of *WT1* expression remain to be dissected, the paired-box gene *PAX2*, which is normally expressed in the Wolffian duct, uteric bud and metanephric mesenchyme, fails to be expressed in the latter in *WT1*-mutant embryos. This suggests that *WT1* may positively regulate *PAX2* expression in the condensing mesenchyme. A role for *WT1* in the regulation of *PAX2* expression was previously predicted from co-localization studies, although at that time it was postulated that *WT1* would exert a negative effect on *PAX2* expression, since as *WT1* expression increased in the maturing glomeruli, *PAX2* expression declined.[21] Obviously, the regulation of these transcription factors is complex and we still do not know if, for example, different isoforms of *WT1* play distinct roles in the developing embryo.

All available evidence suggests that *WT1* is intimately involved in regulating the response of cells to mesenchymal induction of urogenital development. The common localization of *WT1* expression just prior to and including the period of active organogenesis in humans and rodents suggests conservation of function through restriction to specific sites of spatial and temporal expression.[6-9,11,22] The expression pattern of *WT1* is restricted to derivatives of the intermediate and lateral mesoderm, and ectoderm including the kidney, gonads, spleen and serosal membranes lining the body cavities, and in the developing abdominal musculature, and uterus. Other mesodermal derivatives including cartilage, bone, heart, blood cells, lymph vessels and cells, and cortex of the adrenal gland do not express *WT1*. However, the urogenital system appears to be unique in that it is only here that the pattern of *WT1* expression parallels the timing of differentiation within the nephrogenic cord, the three stages of developmental renal formation, the uterus, and the gonadal structures.

It should be noted that the mesodermal derivatives of well-differentiated epithelium such as the renal tubules, the urothelial lining of the collecting system and ureter, and rudimentary nephric, mesonephric and paramesonephric duct structures do not express *WT1*. Remarkably, a specific role for *WT1* in mesenchymal induction of epithelial differentiation is also suggested by studying Wilms tumors themselves. There appears to be a correlation between differential expression of *WT1* and the histopathologic content of various mesenchymal and epithelial components[4] such that higher expression of *WT1* correlates with the presence of a significant (>50%) content of blastema and epithelial derivatives. Further understanding of the role of *WT1* in kidney development awaits the description of downstream targets and upstream regulators of this gene.

REFERENCES

1. Huang A, Campbell CE, Bonetta L, McAndrews-Hill M, Chilton-MacNeill S, Coppes MJ, Law DJ, Feinberg AP, Yeger H, Williams BRG: Tissue, developmental, and tumor-specific expression of divergent transcripts in Wilms tumor. Science 1990; 250:991-994.
2. Call KM, Glaser T, Ito CY, Buckler AJ, Pelletier J, Haber DA, Rose EA, Kral A, Yeger H, Lewis WH, Jones C, Housman DE: Isolation and characterization of a zinc finger polypeptide gene at the human chromosome 11 Wilms' tumor locus. Cell 1990; 60:509-520.

3. Pritchard JK, Fleming S: Cell types expressing the Wilms' tumour gene (WT1) in Wilms' tumours. Oncogene 1991; 6:2211-2220.

4. Yeger H, Cullinane C, Flenniken A, Chilton-MacNeill S, Campbell C, Huang A, Bonetta L, Coppes MJ, Thorner P, Williams BRG: Coordinate expression of Wilms tumor genes correlates with Wilms tumor phenotypes. Cell Growth Differentiation 1992; 3:855-864.

5. Pritchard-Jones K, Fleming S, Davidson D, Bickmore W, Porteous D, Gosden C, Bard J, Buckler A, Pelletier J, Housman D, Van Heyningen V, Hastie N: The candidate Wilms' tumour gene is involved in genitourinary development. Nature 1990; 346:194-197.

6. Pelletier J, Schalling M, Buckler AJ, Rogers A, Haber DA, Housman D: Expression of the Wilms' tumor gene WT1 in the murine urogenital system. Genes Dev 1991; 5:1345-1356.

7. Buckler AJ, Pelletier J, Haber DA, Glaser T, Housman DE: Isolation, characterization, and expression of the murine Wilms' tumor gene (WT1) during kidney development. Mol Cell Biol 1991; 11:1707-1712.

8. Armstrong JF, Pritchard-Jones K, Bickmore WA, Hastie ND, Bard JBL: The expression of the Wilms' tumour gene, WT1, in the developing mammalian embryo. Mechanisms of Development 1993; 40:85-97.

9. Sharma PM, Yang X, Bowman M, Roberts V, Sukumar S: Molecular cloning of rat Wilms tumor complementary DNA and a study of messenger RNA expression in the urogenital system and the brain. Cancer Res 1992; 52:6407-6412.

10. Moore KL: The Developing Human Embryo. Philadelphia: W.B. Saunders Co., 1982.

11. Rackley RR, Flenniken AM, Kuriyan NP, Kessler PM, Stoler MH, Williams BRG: Expression of the Wilms' tumor suppressor gene *WT1* during mouse embryogenesis. Cell Growth Differentiation 1993; 4:1023-1031.

12. Park S, Schalling M, Bernard A, Maheswaran S, Shipley GC, Roberts D, Fletcher J, Shipman R, Rheinwald J, Demetri G, Griffin J, Minden M, Housman DE, Haber DA: The Wilms tumour gene WT1 is expressed in murine mesoderm-derived tissues and mutated in a human mesothelioma. Nature Genetics 1993; 4:415-420.

13. Mundlos S, Pelletier J, Darveau A, Bachmann M, Winterpacht A, Zabel B: Nuclear localization of the protein encoded by the Wilms tumor gene WT1 in embryonic and adult tisuue. Develop 1993; 119:1329-1341.

14. Miwa H, Beran M, Saunders GF: Expression of the Wilms' tumor gene (WT1) in human leukemias. Leukemia 1992; 6:405-409.

15. Inoue K, Sugiyama H, Ogawa H, Nakagawa M, Yamagami T, Miwa H, Kita K, Hiraoka A, Nasu K, Kyo T, Dohy H, Nakauchi H, Ishidate T, Akkiyama T, Kishimoto T: WT1 as a prognostic factor and a new marker for the detection of minimal residual disease. Blood 1994; 84:3071-3079.

16. Phelan SA, Lindberg C, Call KM: Wilms tumor gene, WT1, mRNA is down-regulated during induction of erythroid and megakaryotic differentiation of K562 cells. Cell Growth Differentiation 1994; 5:677-686.

17. Sekiya M, Adachi M, Hinoda Y, Imai K, Yachi A: Downregulation of Wilms' tumor gene (WT1) during myelomonocytic differentiation in HL60 cells. Blood 1994; 83:11876-11882.

18. Kaufman MH: The Atlas of Mouse Development. New York: Academic Press, 1992.

19. Zhou J, Rauscher FJ III, Bondy C: Wilms' tumor (WT1) gene expression in decidual differentiation. Differentiation 1993; 54:109-114.

20. Kreidberg JA, Sarlola H, Loring JM, Maeda M, Pelletier J, Housman D, Jaenish R: WT-1 is required for early kidney development. Cell 1993; 74:679-691.

21. Eccles MR, Wallis LJ, Fidler AE, Spurr NK, Goodfellow PJ, Reeve AE: Expression of *PAX2* gene in human fetal kidney and Wilms tumor. Cell Growth Differentiation 1992; 3:279-289.

22. Pritchard-Jones K, Fleming S: Cell types expressing the Wilms' tumour gene (WT1) in Wilms' tumours: implications for tumour histogenesis. Oncogene 1991; 6:2211-20.

CHAPTER 6

CELLULAR FUNCTIONS OF WT1

INTRODUCTION

Even prior to the cloning of the gene, the genetics and phenotype of Wilms tumors strongly suggested that the function of the WT1 protein would be to act as a tumor suppressor. The implications of this designation are that *WT1* is in some general way involved in regulating either cell cycle control or differentiation, the two processes that are altered in the conversion of normal to transformed cells. Given the tissue and developmentally restricted pattern of expression of *WT1* (see chapter 5), and the phenotype of transgenic mice in which both alleles of the *WT1* gene have been rendered inactive,[1] it is most probable that *WT1* is involved in differentiation. The transgenic null mice exhibit a clear block in kidney differentiation, with development progressing to the stage of metanephric blastemal formation followed by apparent apoptosis at the point where *WT1* expression would be induced in normal mice.[1] Interestingly, even though mesonephric kidney expresses low levels of *WT1* mRNA[2] and protein[3] in normal animals, mesonephric development appears normal in the transgenic null animals.

WT1 IS A DNA BINDING PROTEIN CONTAINING FOUR C2H2 ZINC FINGERS

WT1 is a classic example of a gene whose primary sequence provided strong clues as to its cellular function. The largest open reading frame of the longest *WT1* transcript is 1347 bp and encodes a protein of 449 amino acids (Fig. 6.1). Two alternative splice sites result in four potential isoforms of the protein[4] that differ by the presence or absence of 17 amino acids in the amino terminal domain and the presence or absence of three amino acids

Wilms Tumor: Clinical and Molecular Characterization, by Max J. Coppes, Christine E. Campbell, and Bryan R.G. Williams. © 1995 R.G. Landes Company.

(KTS) in the carboxy terminal domain of the protein. These isoforms will be referred to as WT1+17aa+KTS, WT1-17aa+KTS, WT1+17aa-KTS, WT1-17aa-KTS. The first alternative splice site removes amino acids 250 to 266, while the second removes amino acids 408-410. The protein consists of an amino terminal proline and glutamine-rich domain and a carboxy terminal domain consisting of four homologous zinc finger motifs of the C2H2 class. The amino terminal proline/glutamine rich domain is characteristic of many transactivation domains of transcriptional factors,[5] while the carboxy zinc finger motif is characteristic of a DNA binding domain.

THE DNA BINDING DOMAIN OF *WT1*

Zinc fingers are one of the most common and best characterized protein motifs. There are several different classes of zinc fingers depending upon the amino acids involved in coordination of the zinc ion. The C2H2 class consists of proteins in which the zinc ion is coordinated by two cysteine (Cys) and two histidine (His) residues whose spacing is highly conserved. The signature sequence of C2H2 zinc fingers as defined by the PROSITE database is C-X(2,4)-C-X(12)-H-X(3,5)-H where X is any amino acid. In addition to the conservation of spacing between the Cys and His residues, the spacing between adjacent functional zinc fingers tends to be highly conserved to the extent that degenerate oligonucleotides corresponding to this amino acid sequence have been utilized to isolate novel zinc finger encoding genes.[6-8] Proteins containing C2H2 zinc finger motifs include some RNA binding proteins (e.g. ref. 9) but the majority are site-specific DNA binding proteins.[10] Within a single protein, C2H2 zinc fingers may be present in anywhere from a few copies to, for example, the 37 copies found in the Xenopus Xfin protein.[9] There is some evidence that within proteins containing multiple zinc finger motifs there may also be non-functional zinc fingers that have lost one or more of the Cys or His residues presumably necessary for metal ion coordination. Some zinc finger-containing proteins exhibit alternative splicing leading to the synthesis of protein isoforms consisting of different subsets of zinc fingers.[10] This results in proteins with distinct DNA binding specificities. The crystal structures of several zinc finger DNA binding peptides have been solved in recent years including a co-crystal of the EGR1 or zif268 DNA

Fig. 6.1. Amino acid sequence of WT1. Two alternatively spliced sequences are indicated in boldface uppercase letters. The four zinc fingers are underlined with the "linker regions" between them indicated in italics. Amino acids Gly201, Ser273, Leu281 and Ser365 which are referred to in the text are indicated in boldface.

```
Met Gly Ser Asp Val Arg Asp Leu Asn Ala Leu Leu Pro Ala Val Pro Ser   17
Leu Gly Gly Gly Gly Gly Cys Ala Leu Pro Val Ser Gly Ala Ala Gln Trp   34
Ala Pro Val Leu Asp Phe Ala Pro Pro Gly Ala Ser Ala Tyr Gly Ser Leu   51
Gly Gly Pro Ala Pro Pro Pro Ala Pro Pro Pro Pro Pro Pro Pro Pro Pro   68
His Ser Phe Ile Lys Gln Glu Pro Ser Trp Gly Gly Ala Glu Pro His Glu   85
Glu Gln Cys Leu Ser Ala Phe Thr Val His Phe Ser Gly Gln Phe Thr Gly  102
Thr Ala Gly Ala Cys Arg Tyr Gly Pro Phe Gly Pro Pro Pro Pro Ser Gln  119
Ala Ser Ser Gly Gln Ala Arg Met Phe Pro Asn Ala Pro Tyr Leu Pro Ser  136
Cys Leu Glu Ser Gln Pro Ala Ile Arg Asn Gln Gly Tyr Ser Thr Val Thr  153
Phe Asp Gly Thr Pro Ser Tyr Gly His Thr Pro Ser His His Ala Ala Gln  170
Phe Pro Asn His Ser Phe Lys His Glu Asp Pro Met Gly Gln Gln Gly Ser  187
Leu Gly Glu Gln Gln Tyr Ser Val Pro Pro Pro Val Tyr **Gly** Cys His Thr  204
Pro Thr Asp Ser Cys Thr Gly Ser Gln Ala Leu Leu Leu Arg Thr Pro Tyr  221
Ser Ser Asp Asn Leu Tyr Gln Met Thr Ser Gln Leu Glu Cys Met Thr Trp  238
Asn Gln Met Asn Leu Gly Ala Thr Leu Lys Gly **VAL ALA ALA GLY SER SER**  255
**SER SER VAL LYS TRP THR GLU THR GLY GLN SER ASN** His Ser Thr Gly Tyr Glu  272
**Ser** Asp Asn His Thr Thr Pro Ile **Leu** Cys Gly Ala Gln Tyr Arg Ile His  289
Thr His Gly Val Phe Arg Gly Ile Gln Asp Val Arg Arg Val Pro Gly Val  306
Ala Pro Thr Leu Val Arg Ser Ala Ser Glu Thr Ser Glu Lys Arg Pro Phe  323
Met Cys Ala Tyr Pro Gly Cys Asn Lys Arg Tyr Phe Lys Leu Ser His Leu  340
Gln Met His Ser Arg Lys His *Thr Gly* Glu Lys Pro Tyr Gln Cys Asp Phe  357
Lys Asp Cys Glu Arg Arg Phe **Ser** Arg Ser Asp Gln Leu Lys Arg His Gln  374
Arg Arg His *Thr Gly* Val Lys Pro Phe Gln Cys Lys Thr Cys Gln Arg **Lys**  391
Phe Ser Arg Ser Asp His Leu Lys Thr His Thr Arg Thr His *Thr Gly* **LYS**  408
**THR SER** Glu Lys Pro Phe Ser Cys Arg Trp Pro Ser Cys Gln Lys Lys Phe  425
Ala Arg Ser Asp Glu Leu Val Arg His His Asn Met His Gln Arg Asn Met  442
Thr Lys Leu Gln Leu Ala Leu
```

binding domain with a cognate oligonucleotide.[11] A comparison of the crystal structures of two other zinc finger proteins[11,12] with that of EGR1 has demonstrated that not all zinc fingers interact with DNA in exactly the same way. However, as EGR1 is the most highly homologous protein to WT1, its structure is likely the most relevant. The results of the structural analysis of EGR1[11] indicated that the protein fits within the major groove of the DNA with each of the three zinc fingers interacting with three contiguous nucleotides. The amino acid base contacts involve arginine (Arg) or His interactions with guanine residues (Fig. 6.2). This structure was highly satisfying as it explains how DNA binding specificity can be altered by combing different zinc fingers and has resulted in several attempts to alter DNA binding affinity and/ or specificity by mutation of specific amino acids within the DNA binding domain.[13-15]

In the case of EGR1, fingers 1 and 3, which are most highly homologous to each other, are involved in identical base contacts and recognize the sequence 5'-GNG (where N is any nucleotide), while finger 2 makes slightly different contacts and recognizes 5'-NGG. Reading along the G rich strand, the carboxy terminal zinc finger recognizes the 5' end of the oligonucleotide while the amino terminal finger interacts with the 3' end of the oligonucleotide. The crystal structure also indicated the relative orientation of each finger with respect to the DNA is quite similar. This latter observation suggests that the "linker" regions between adjacent zinc fingers may be important in orienting the protein. In this regard, it is interesting to note that one of the two alternative splice sites of WT1 results in the insertion of three amino acids into the linker region between zinc fingers 3 and 4 (WT1 isoforms +17aa+KTS or -17aa+KTS, Fig. 6.1).

The hypothesis that WT1 is a DNA binding protein has been confirmed by a number of laboratories beginning with the work of Rauscher and colleagues. They initially demonstrated that the zinc finger domain of WT1, synthesized as a recombinant protein in *E. coli*, could be immobilized on Sepharose and used to select from random oligonucleotides those that bound with high affinity to the recombinant protein.[16] The results of this experiment demonstrated that the sequence specificity of one form of the WT1 DNA binding domain was very similar to that of several other C2H2 zinc finger proteins, namely those of the early growth re-

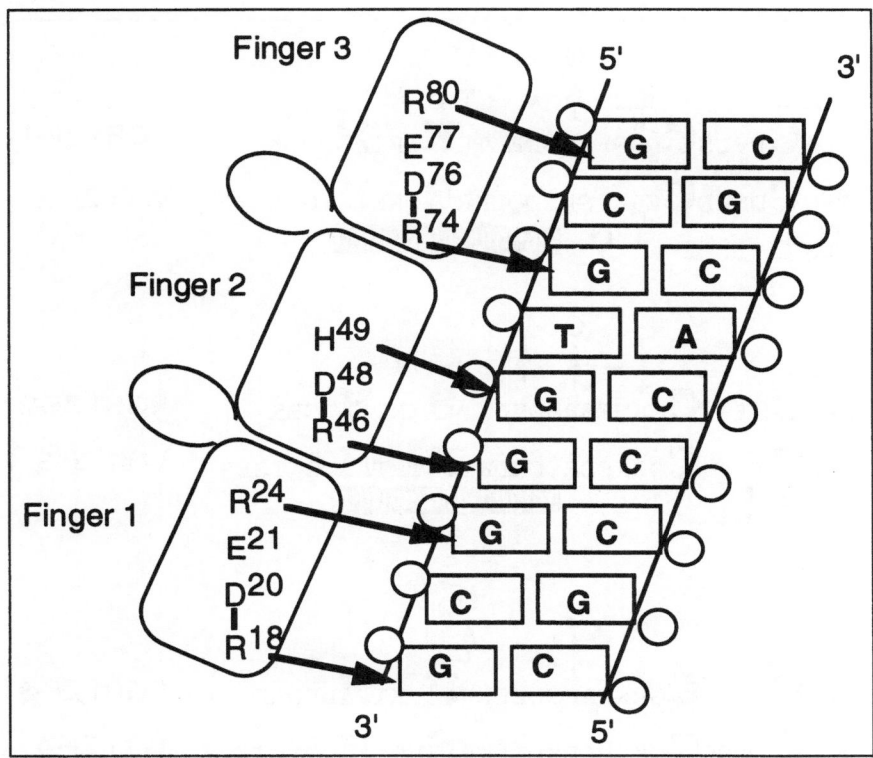

Fig. 6.2. A schematic diagram of the amino acid-base contacts made by EGR1 with a cognate oligonucleotide. Note that positions -1 (i.e., R18, R46 and R74), +3 (i.e., H49) and +6 (R24 and R80) with respect to the first amino acid of the a helix are important for base contacts. A conserved aspartic acid at position +2 (D20, D48 and D76) interacts with the Arg at -1 and stabilizes its base contact.

sponse factor or EGR family. The first member of this family to be cloned was EGR1 (also referred to in the literature as Zif268, Krox-24 or NGFI-A). A search of the protein databases with the WT1 protein sequence indicates that the sequence similarity between WT1 and EGR1 within their DNA binding domains is stronger than between WT1 and any other protein. Zinc fingers 2-4 of WT1 and the three zinc fingers of EGR1 exhibit 55-75% sequence identity within individual zinc finger motifs. In particular, all of the amino acids shown to be involved in protein/DNA contacts in EGR1[11] are conserved in WT1 (Fig. 6.3). Indeed WT1 is sometimes referred to as a member of the EGR1-like family of zinc finger proteins. This is probably somewhat misleading since the genomic organization of the WT1 gene is very different from

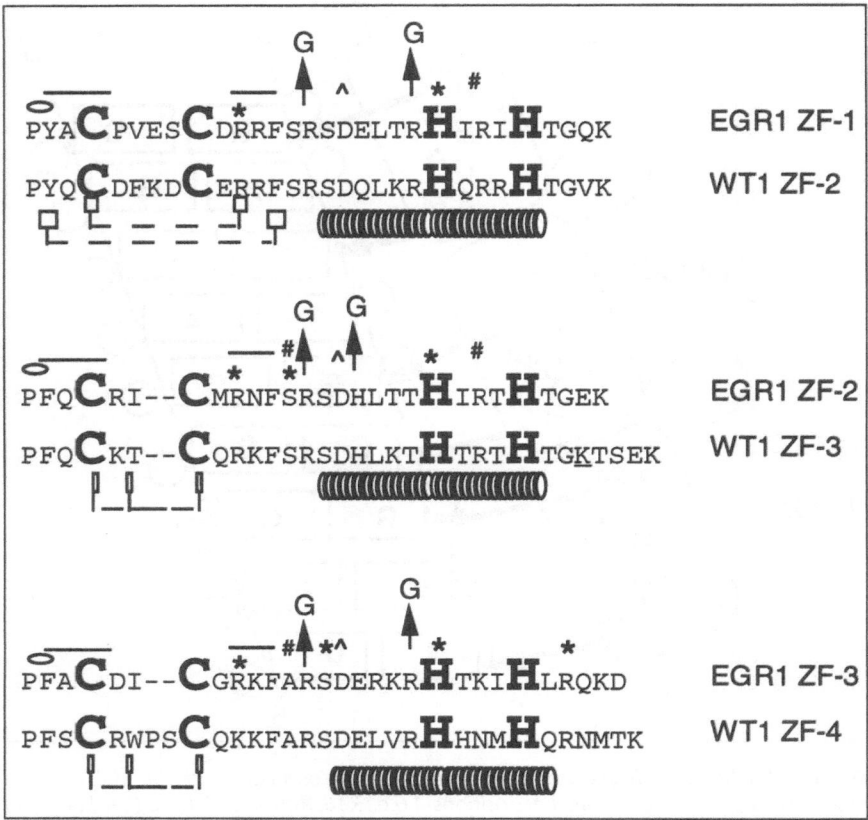

Fig. 6.3. (Continued on facing page)

other EGR1-like family members (such as EGR2 and EGR3). The three zinc fingers of EGR1 and related family members EGR2, EGR3 and pAT133 are encoded by a single exon[17-20] while each of the four zinc fingers of WT1 is encoded by a separate exon. This latter exon organization provides the opportunity for alternative splicing to produce multiple proteins with different DNA binding domains, each with slightly different DNA binding specificity. Although WT1 does direct the synthesis of alternatively spliced transcripts as discussed below, there is no evidence that alternative splicing involves the exclusion of entire zinc fingers from the products. However, there has been a recent report[21] that a subset of desmoplastic small round cell tumors carry a chimeric gene consisting of the 5' end of the *EWS* gene fused to the eighth exon of *WT1*. This gene has the coding capacity to direct the synthesis of

Fig. 6.3. Conservation between EGR1 and WT1 of amino acids important in determining DNA binding.

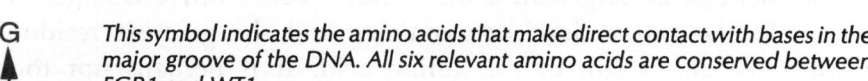 indicates portion of each zinc finger which folds into an α-helical structure.

——   indicates antiparallel β-sheet protein structure.

C C H H These are the Cys and His residues involved in coordinating the zinc ion. Note that all six Cys and His residues are conserved between EGR1 and WT1.

G   This symbol indicates the amino acids that make direct contact with bases in the major groove of the DNA. All six relevant amino acids are conserved between EGR1 and WT1.

*   indicates contacts with the phosphodiester oxygen in the DNA. Eight out of nine of these amino acids are conserved between EGR1 and WT1.

^   This indicates the aspartic acid (D) residue in each zinc finger that stabilizes the contact between Arg (R) and a guanine (G). The three relevant Asp residues are conserved between EGR1 and WT1.

o   indicates a proline and an aromatic amino acid (phenylalanine F or tyrosine Y) that interact in each of the zinc fingers of the EGR1 protein and are also present in the corresponding zinc fingers of WT1.

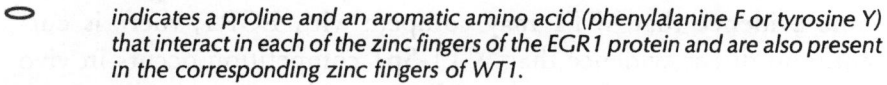 The amino acids indicated are part of the β-sheet structure of each zinc finger and are involved in hydrogen bonding amongst themselves. These amino acids are conserved between the first finger of EGR1 and the second finger of WT1 (i.e., Y and F and C and R of EGR1). However in zinc finger 3 of WT1 a threonine (T) replaces an isoleucine (I), and in zinc finger 4 of WT1 a tryptophane (W) replaces an isoleucine.

indicates contacts between the arginine (R) residue of one finger and a serine (S) or alanine (A) of the next. Both the R residues and the S or A residues are conserved between EGR1 and WT1.

a fusion protein in which the RNA binding domain of the EWS protein is replaced by three of the four zinc fingers of the DNA binding domain of WT1. The functional relevance of this fusion protein to the phenotype of those tumors is unknown, although one might expect the resulting protein to be involved in transcriptional activation or repression.

One significant difference between WT1 and EGR1 is the presence of an additional zinc finger in the former with respect to the latter. The first zinc finger of WT1 has the least sequence homology with any of the zinc fingers of EGR1 although it most closely resembles zinc finger 2 in terms of potential amino acid-base contacts. However, the first zinc finger of WT1 is more like the first zinc finger of another family of C2H2 site specific DNA binding proteins, the Sp1 family, and in particular Sp3, one member of this family[10,22] (Fig. 6.4). In particular, the second Arg that is involved in contacting the third base of the triplet in EGR1 zinc finger 2 (i.e., R46 in Fig. 6.2), is replaced in Sp3 and WT1 with a Lysine (Lys) residue. It should be noted that in this context, replacement of an Arg with a Lys is not a conservative change, as the molecular interactions between Arg and the guanine residue involve the side chain of the amino acid. It is perhaps not too surprising that, although both EGR1 and Sp1 proteins bind to GC rich sequences their binding specificities do not overlap.[10] This raises the possibility that the in vivo targets of WT1 are not EGR1-like sequences, but related sequences. It also suggests that WT1 may function through competitive or possibly cooperative interactions with both EGR1 and Sp1 binding sites. Although there is some evidence that WT1 may compete with EGR1, there is currently no direct evidence that WT1-Sp1 competition occurs in vivo in transient transfection assays. However, there is a recent report (described below) that WT1 may bind to Sp1-like binding sites and inhibit DNA replication from the SV40 origin. Moreover, it has been noted that some of the natural promoters to which WT1 can bind in DNase protection assays have overlapping WT1/EGR1 and Sp1 binding sites[23] so that binding of one protein would likely sterically inhibit binding of the other. To further complicate the issue of WT1 binding specificity, some WT1 binding sites that are not consensus EGR1 binding sites have been identified.[24]

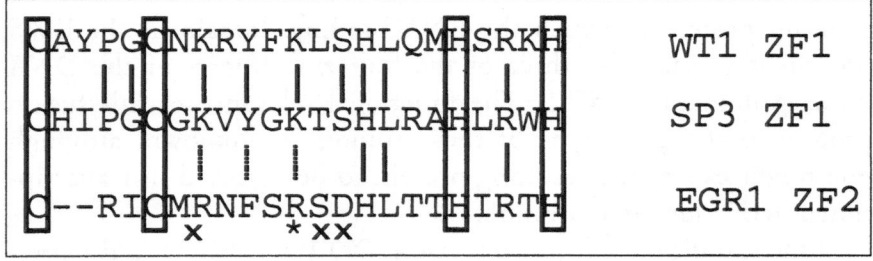

Fig. 6.4. A comparison of the first zinc finger of WT1 with the first zinc finger of Sp3 and the second zinc finger of EGR1. Homology is indicated by solid vertical lines. Note that in addition to Arg46 (indicated with an *) that is involved in an amino acid-base contact, several other of the important amino acids identified in Figure 6.3 in this figure are not present in the first zinc finger of WT1 or Sp3 (i.e., the R and S residues involved in contacting phosphodiester oxygen and the D that stabilizes the arginine-guanine contact).

A summary of WT1 binding sites identified to date is presented in Figure 6.5.

Unlike many DNA binding proteins, such as nuclear factor I or Ap1,[10] there is no evidence that WT1 binds to DNA in any form larger than a monomer. It has been noted by several authors however that WT1 does include a putative leucine-zipper-like sequence[30] that could contribute to WT1 homo- or hetero-dimerization.

WT1 INHIBITS T AG AND SV40 ORIGIN DEPENDENT REPLICATION

Recently, it has been reported[30] that expression of either the +KTS or -KTS isoforms of WT1 inhibits replication of plasmids containing SV40 origins. In this experiment the SV40 origin was on the same plasmid as the CMV promoter driving expression of *WT1*. Although plasmids containing full-length *WT1* (either +KTS or -KTS) were the least efficiently replicated in this assay, plasmids directing the synthesis of full-length *EGR1* or truncated *WT1* containing plasmids also had an effect, making it difficult to interpret

EGRI consensus binding sites	Non- consensus binding sites
GCGGGGGCG [2]	GAGGGGGTC [7]
GATCTACGAGAGGGAGGATACTTAC [4]	CGAGGGGCA [7]
GAGTGGGTG [7]	GAGGGGCGG [7]
	CTGGGGAGG [7]
	G**GAGAGG**AGGAGGAGGA [1]
	TGTGTGTGTGTGTGTGTGTGTGTGTGT [3]
	AGAGGAGGGTGTCT [6]
	AGCAGGGGGAGGCT [6]
	TTTGGAGGGAGGGGCAGGTAGGCTCTAG [5]

Fig. 6.5. WT1 binding sites. WT1 binding sites are separated into consensus EGR1 binding sites (i.e., 5'- GNGNGGGNG-3') and non-consensus sites that differ at one or more positions from the consensus site. 1) Identified in the PDGF A chain promoter as binding the -KTS form of WT1.[25] 2) EGR1 consensus binding sequence that binds -KTS forms of WT1 and is found in the context of the EGR1,[26] IGF2,[27] PDGF A chain[28,29] and CSF[23] promoters. 3) Oligonucleotide identified as binding -KTS forms of WT1.[24] 4) Oligonucleotide identified as binding +KTS or -KTS forms of WT1.[24] 5) Oligonucleotide identified by Yee et al, (manuscript in preparation) as binding +KTS or -KTS forms of WT1. 6) DNA sequence derived from WT1 promoter identified as binding +KTS or -KTS forms of WT1 by methylation interference. 7) Oligonucleotides originally identified by Rauscher et al,[16] as binding WT1-KTS.

these results. Nonetheless, it was possible to show that replication inhibition required both the DNA binding domain and amino acids 67-180 of the N terminal transcriptional regulatory domain. It was also shown that this effect required the 21bp repeats of the SV40 origin and that bacterially-expressed recombinant *WT1* DNA binding domains, either with or without the KTS insertion, were capable of binding to the GC-rich 21 bp repeat sequence in a gel mobility shift assay. The authors were unable to detect any stable association between the SV40 T Ag and WT1 proteins using immunoprecipitation. These data suggest that WT1 may be yet another example of a transcriptional regulatory factor that also functions in viral DNA replication. The best studied examples of such factors are probably nuclear factor I and Oct-1, both of which play a stimulatory role in the replication of adenovirus.[31,32] Although this report has yet to be confirmed, it raises the interesting possibility that WT1 might also play a role in cellular DNA replication and that inhibition of cellular replication could be a component of its function as a tumor suppressor gene.

WT1 IS AN UNUSUAL C2H2 ZINC FINGER PROTEIN

Although there is no evidence for differential splicing resulting in utilization of different subsets of zinc fingers (at least in wild-type protein), WT1 has an interesting unique feature among the approximately 200 zinc finger proteins currently in the PROSITE database. One of the two alternative splice sites of WT1 inserts three amino acids (KTS) into the highly-conserved linker region[10] between two adjacent zinc fingers. This insertion, based on the cocrystalization data of Pavletich et al,[11] would not perturb the structure of the zinc finger but may perturb the spacing between adjacent fingers. As expected, the isoforms of WT1 that include the three amino acid insertion (+KTS) bind very poorly to some EGR1 or WT1-KTS binding sites but bind almost as well as WT1-KTS to others. This may indicate that the four zinc fingers of WT1 contribute unequally and differently to binding to different sites. Thus, even though the KTS insertion might make it difficult to orient the fourth zinc finger of the +KTS form of WT1 into the major groove of the DNA, if this finger is contributing little to the overall binding affinity to that particular DNA sequence, then one would not expect WT1-KTS and WT1+KTS to exhibit different binding properties. Alternatively, differences in the higher order structure or flexibility of the DNA itself that will result from differences in sequence may be more or less accommodating of the KTS insertion in the linker region of the protein. The relative abundance of the four transcripts among tissues that express WT1 is highly conserved,[4] strongly suggesting that all forms of WT1 play a role in the normal function of the protein. Furthermore, a report by Haber et al[33] demonstrating that all four isoforms of WT1 are capable individually of causing growth suppression of a Wilms tumor cell line supports the hypothesis that the +KTS forms of the protein have a function independent of the -KTS forms. The physiological significance of multiple isoforms of WT1 remains to be determined, but in addition to the presence of all four among all mammalian cells expressing WT1, the ability to synthesize at least the +KTS and -KTS isoforms is evolutionarily conserved in chickens and alligators.[34]

WT1 IS A TRANSCRIPTIONAL REGULATOR

The ability of the WT1-KTS DNA binding domain to bind to EGR1-like sequences and the presence of a transcription factor-like proline/glutamine rich amino terminal domain, are reflected in transient transfection experiments which have demonstrated that WT1-KTS can repress or induce the transcription of reporter constructs depending upon the placement of the EGR1 like sequences within the promoter.[26-29,35-37] Transcriptional activity is also modulated by the presence of functional p53 protein.[38] The first of these reports[26] demonstrated that transfection of expression vectors directing the expression of WT1-17aa-KTS or WT1+17aa-KTS repressed transcription from the EGR1 promoter driving CAT by 9-fold in 3T3 cells. WT1+KTS isoforms or deletion mutants that removed either the DNA binding domain or part of the N-terminal domain had no effect. A more recent report[38] suggests that in the absence of functional p53, both WT1+KTS and WT1-KTS isoforms will activate transcription from the EGR1 promoter in Saos-2 cells, but the -KTS isoform does so more efficiently (~40X vs 5X for +KTS). In this experiment, adding back wild-type p53 by cotransfection with a p53 expression vector reduced the activation from ~40X to 9X but did not result in repression as had been described previously. This observation suggests that the transcriptional regulatory function of WT1 may be modulated in a cell-specific manner.

In this regard, Madden et al[39] found that WT1-GAL4 fusion proteins act as repressors of transcription more efficiently in 3T3 than in 293 cells. WT1 can suppress *IGF2* in HepG2 cells by ~10X, again demonstrated by utilizing transient transfection to introduce *WT1* into the cells.[27] A control expression construct directing the synthesis of a truncated protein had no effect. WT1 can also suppress human platelet-derived growth factor A chain in NIH3T3 cells up to 50X.[28] Again, a truncated protein had no effect. These researchers also showed that the PDGF A promoter contained multiple WT1 binding sites. Further analysis of the PDGF A chain promoter[29,35] demonstrated that WT1 can activate as well as suppress in NIH3T3 or 293 cells (adenovirus transformed kidney epithelial cells) depending upon how much of the promoter sequence is present. The region from -153 to +388 suppressed (<50X) while that from -60 to +388 activated (4X). These investigators also found that deleting from +14 to +105 would activate chimeric gene constructs, suggesting that the presence of both 5' and 3' WT1 binding sites is necessary for repression while deletion of one or the other resulted in activation. The first 84 amino acids of WT1 which include the highly proline-rich domain could be deleted without affecting activity. However, deletion of the first 178 amino acids of WT1 resulted in a protein that could still activate transcription but could no longer repress. This is consistent with the results of Madden et al[26] who found that deletion of the first 178 amino acids resulted in a protein that failed to repress the EGR1 promoter. In the case of the PDGF A chain promoter, activation still required the presence of only 5' or 3' sites. In the presence of both 5' and 3' WT1 binding sites, this mutant had no effect. Using similar assays, Werner et al[40] showed that IGF1R is repressed by WT1 in CHO cells with the rat promoter being repressed 5X, and the human promoter ~2X.

Several reports have indicated that WT1 may act through binding to sequences other than EGR1 consensus binding sites. Thus, the CSF1 promoter is repressed by WT1 3-4X in fibroblasts or WEHI cells.[23] Moreover, WT1 apparently binds to sites that in the absence of the protein are bound by Sp1 and Sp3. This latter observation was based on the ability of antibodies against the Sp1 or Sp3 proteins to alter the mobility of protein/DNA complexes in non-denaturing acrylamide gels (electrophoretic mobility shift or band-shift assays). It has also been reported that a second WT1 binding sequence in the PDGF A chain promoter that is not obviously EGR1-like but also binds EGR1 and WT1, can function in transient transfection assays in NIH3T3 cells.[35]

Although most of the original studies were carried out with constructs expressing one of the two WT1-KTS forms of the protein, several more recent studies have shown that WT1+KTS isoforms can also affect transcription. Rupprech et al[41] reported that WT1 protein suppresses its own promoter in 293 cells. In this assay either WT1+KTS or WT1-KTS isoforms were functional. This was not first report that +KTS forms of WT1 could bind DNA[24] but was the first to show that WT1+KTS could function in a transient transfection assay, in this case suppressing transcription from a chimeric construct driven by -513 to +254 of its own promoter. Interestingly, repression was greatly enhanced in the +KTS isoform by the presence of the 17 amino acids encoded by alternatively spliced exon 5. No difference in transcriptional modulation was seen between WT1-17aa -KTS and WT1+17aa -KTS. To support their transient transfection data, Rupprech et al demonstrated by a combination of DNase footprinting and methylation interference that both +KTS and -KTS forms of WT1 can bind to DNA. DNA contacts were identical for at least one oligonucleotide tested but differed for a second. The DNase footprinting experiments also suggest that WT1 contacts a larger site than EGR1, consistent with the presence of an additional zinc finger. The importance of this first zinc finger to the function of the WT1 protein is supported by the report of a missence mutation in the first finger in a Denys-Drash patient.[42] Drummond et al[43] have demonstrated that WT1+KTS can also bind to the P3 and P4 promoters of IGF2 and repress transcription from chimeric genes that include these sequences. As with the previous report the +KTS +17aa form of the protein appeared to interact with a subset of the sites that interact with the -KTS forms of the protein. To date, no binding sites specific for the +KTS form of the protein have been reported. However, Drummond and co-workers made two additional interesting observations with respect to the DNA binding of WT1. The first, based on methylation interference and gel mobility shift assays with different oligonucleotide probes, was that the WT1 zinc finger domain may interact with DNA in a modular fashion with some binding sites requiring all four zinc fingers while others may utilize only three. The second observation was that a tumor associated *WT1* mutation that results in the in frame deletion of the entire third zinc finger was capable of binding to both a subset of sequences bound by wild-type WT1 proteins and to a unique sequence not bound by other WT1 isoforms. Interestingly, this mutation is found in a heterozygous state in tumor tissue,[44] suggesting that it may act in a dominant fashion. These data[43] provide a possible explanation for this observation; namely that the mutant protein may exert its phenotypic effect through its ability to regulate genes not normally regulated by WT1 or by interfering with wild-type protein function through competitively binding to a subset of WT1 binding sites.

Mutant WT1 proteins have also provided some interesting data regarding the question of what controls whether WT1 functions as an activator or repressor of transcription. The same single amino acid alteration (Gly 201 -> Asp) found in a Wilms tumor was inserted into a CMV driven murine *WT1* expression construct.[45] The resultant construct was cotransfected with an EGR1-CAT reporter construct into NIH3T3 cells. Whereas the wild-type protein repressed CAT expression by ~4-fold from the EGR1 promoter, the mutant caused a 6-fold activation of the same construct. A similar effect was observed with a second mutation in the *WT1* gene that was found in a human mesothelioma.[45] In this case Ser273 was converted to a glycine and, again inserting this into an expression construct, resulted in transcriptional activation of an EGR1-CAT reporter construct.

In speculating about the function of the first zinc finger, it is worth noting that this zinc finger has more sequence homology to one of the SP3 zinc fingers than to any of the EGR1 zinc fingers (see Fig. 6.2). It should be noted that the binding specificities of SP3 and EGR1, although they both recognize GC rich oligonucleotides are very different. This raises the possibility that despite the ability of the protein to bind to EGR1-like sites in vitro, and to repress transcription of promoters containing EGR1-like sites in transient transfection assays, at least some of the genes that are targets of regulation by the WT1 protein may not contain EGR1-like DNA binding sites and will therefore only be identified using a procedure that does not specifically look for the presence of such sites in the gene promoter. Transient transfection assays result in levels of protein expression within transfected cells that are much higher than those normally found in vivo. This may result in WT1 binding in transient transfection assays to sites which it fails to bind in vivo because of competition with other proteins.

Taken together, the results of the transient transfection assays suggest that WT1 may bind to sites other than EGR1 consensus binding sites and may function as either a transcriptional repressor or enhancer depending upon the specific promoter, the cell type and the presence of other transcriptional regulatory proteins. This conclusion reemphasizes the need to identify endogenous targets of WT1 in the cells in which it is normally expressed (i.e., differentiating glomerular epithelial cells).

POSSIBLE DOWNSTREAM TARGETS OF WT1 TRANSCRIPTIONAL REGULATION

The genes identified as potential targets of the -KTS forms of the protein based on the transient transfection assays include IGF2,[27] IGF-1R,[36,40] CSF-1,[23] the A chain of PDGF[28] and TGFβ.[46] However, it remains to be demonstrated that the regulation of some of these genes is directly relevant to the normal cellular function of WT1. In interpreting the transient transfection assays thus far reported, the following caveats must be kept in mind. First, the nature of the assay dictates that cells are grossly overexpressing WT1. The second problem with this assay is that transcriptional activity is being directed by a promoter fragment that has been inserted into a plasmid and thereby removed from the context of the remainder of the chromosome. Thus WT1 is probably capable of interacting with the sequences defined by these transient transfection assays but whether these interactions are physiologically relevant remains to be demonstrated. To date no endogenous targets of WT1 regulation have been identified. However, at least two of the genes identified as potential targets by transient transfection assays, IGF-1R[40] and IGF2,[47] are overexpressed in Wilms tumors relative to age matched normal kidneys. Recently the *nov* proto-oncogene has also been suggested as a potential target of WT1 regulation based on an observed inverse correlation between levels of *WT1* and levels of *nov* mRNA in Wilms tumors.[48] However, the heterogeneous histology of Wilms tumors (see chapter 2) makes it difficult to interpret these data. The identification of endogenous targets of WT1 regulation will be important, not only in confirming that WT1 is a transcription factor, but also in understanding why loss of function of this gene leads to the development of Wilms tumor. In addition, it may provide an assay for WT1 function in Wilms tumors.

PROTEIN-PROTEIN INTERACTIONS INVOLVING WT1

To date, the only cellular protein shown to interact with WT1, based on co-immunoprecipitation studies, is the ubiquitously-expressed tumor suppressor p53.[38] The presence of wild-type p53 appears to alter the transcriptional regulatory activity of WT1 so that in the absence of wild-type p53 protein, WT1 will activate transcription from the EGR1 promoter, while in its presence WT1 serves as a transcriptional repressor. This was shown by transient transfection assays of vectors directing the expression of WT1 plus or minus p53 into Saos-2 (lack endogenous p53) or of WT1 alone into rat embryo fibroblasts stably transfected with a temperature-sensitive p53 mutant. Apparently some mutant p53 proteins will also associate with WT1 although they do not alter the transcriptional regulatory properties of WT1.

In addition, there has been a report that a mutant WT1 may cooperate with E1A in transforming BHK cells[49] but in this case no direct evidence of a protein-protein interaction was reported.

OTHER FACTORS THAT MAY CONTRIBUTE TO OR MODIFY THE CELLULAR FUNCTION OF WT1

RNA EDITING

Recently WT1 has been shown to be one of a select few nuclear mammalian genes whose transcripts are subjected to editing. In the case of WT1, editing has been shown to occur in rat kidney and human testes.[50] RNA editing may be generally defined as any modification of the RNA that alters its sequence. In the case of WT1, editing involves a U>C change that alters amino acid 281 (or 280 of the rat) from Leu to Pro (Leu is indicated in bold face in Fig. 6.1). Editing appears to be highly developmentally regulated with very few of the fetal rat kidney transcripts being edited to ~30% of adult rat transcripts carrying the altered sequence.[50] It should be noted that although WT1 is edited in adult rat kidney and in human testes, there is no evidence for editing in human adult kidney. It is possible that editing of WT1 may use at least one of the same subunits as the editing complex of apolipoprotein

B. In this latter case it has also been found that mRNA for the catalytic component of the editing complex is present in adult rat kidney[51] but not in human kidney,[52] although it is present in human testes.[52] To date, neither the enzyme responsible for RNA editing nor its significance as it applies to WT1 are known. It has been shown however, using transient transfection assays, that editing as it occurs in the adult rat kidney may alter the transcriptional regulatory properties of WT1.[50]

PHOSPHORYLATION OF WT1

The functional activity of many transcription factors, including several zinc finger proteins, is altered by phosphorylation. The WT1 protein includes many potential phosphorylation sites for both tyrosine and serine/threonine kinases including a potential serine/threonine kinase site generated by the second alternative splice site of WT1 that results in the insertion of three amino acids (KTS) into the DNA binding domain. Morris et al[53] originally reported that WT1 expressed in transiently, transfected cos cells was not phosphorylated. However, a more recent report by Sharma et al[54] cites a communication that states WT1 is phosphorylated and indicates Ser364 (Ser365 in human WT1, see Fig. 6.1) as a particular amino acid subject to in vivo phosphorylation. Serine 365 is within the DNA binding domain of the protein and thus this report raises the possibility that phosphorylation might alter DNA binding properties of WT1. This particular serine is a potential casein kinase II or cAMP/cGMP responsive kinase phosphorylation target based on the signature sequences of such targets as defined in the PROSITE database. There is at least one other serine within the DNA binding domain in a very similar environment with respect to surrounding amino acids that might also be a potential phosphorylation site. Both of these serines are conserved in EGR1 and the second serine in particular has been shown by Pavletich[11] to participate in an interaction with an arginine residue from the preceding zinc finger (Fig. 6.2). The EGR1 equivalent of Ser365 which is present in the first zinc finger of EGR1 does not interact with the DNA backbone of the binding site but the equivalent serine in the third zinc finger of EGR1 does. This latter serine makes a contact with a phosphate residue on the non-G rich strand of the cognate oligonucleotide. If Ser365 of WT1 makes a similar contact, clearly phosphorylation would perturb such an interaction. This hypothesis remains to be tested.

REDOX REGULATION OF ZINC FINGER PROTEINS

Another potential mechanism for regulating the DNA binding activity of the WT1 protein is through changes in the intracellular oxidation state (redox state). Several important cellular processes have been associated with changes in intracellular redox state including cytokine activation of HIV replication,[55,56] expression of cellular adhesion molecules,[57] aging[58] and apoptotic cell death.[59,60] Also, direct modification of redox state by oxidant or antioxidant treatment has been shown to modulate gene expression.[61-63] Redox regulation of DNA binding activity was first demonstrated with the OxyR protein of *E. coli* where oxidation is required for transcriptional activation by the protein on specific promoter sites.[64-66] Subsequent studies in eukaryotic cells have shown that the DNA binding activity of several different classes of DNA binding proteins including zinc finger proteins EGR1[67] and Sp1[68] is sensitive to oxidative inactivation in vitro. These affects appear to be mediated through the cysteine residues that are involved in coordinating the zinc ion (the relevant residues of WT1 are amino acids 325 and 330 in zinc finger 1, 355 and 360 in the second zinc finger, 385 and 388 in the third zinc finger and amino acids 416 and 421 in the third zinc finger, Fig. 6.1). The ability of a cellular protein, Ref-1[69] to increase the DNA binding activity of EGR1[67] raises the possibility that redox regulation plays a role in modulating the DNA binding activity of this protein in vivo. By extension, given the high degree of conservation between the DNA binding domains of EGR1 and WT1, it is possible that redox-state also modulates WT1 DNA binding activity.

WT1 AND APOPTOSIS

In the last several years it has become very clear that a regulated form of cell death, referred to as apoptosis, plays an important role in embryonic development and in response to DNA damage. In transgenic mice homozygous for a WT1 gene knockout,[1] apoptosis of the kidney blastema occurs at a time in development when normally WT1 expression would be increasing and the mesenchymal derived blastema would be undergoing induction by the ureteric bud into the epithelium of the glomerulus, proximal and distal tubules. This suggests a possible role for WT1 in apoptosis. Additional indirect support for this suggestion may be found in a recently published report that the *bcl2* gene, that encodes a protein known to play an important role in apoptosis, contains a putative WT1 binding site within its second exon.[70] To date however there is no evidence that WT1 actually modulates *bcl2* expression.

CONCLUSION

Although much has been published concerning the role of WT1 as a site-specific DNA binding protein and transcriptional regulator, a great deal remains to be learned. In particular, we still do not know why WT1 exists in four isoforms and we have yet to identify endogenous downstream targets of regulation by WT1. Moreover, we are just beginning to explore possible post-transcriptional modifications that may influence WT1 functional activity.

REFERENCES

1. Kreidberg JA, Sarlola H, Loring JM, Maeda M, Pelletier J, Housman D, Jaenish R: WT-1 is required for early kidney development. Cell 1993; 74:679-691.
2. Rackley RR, Flenniken AM, Kuriyan NP, Kessler PM, Stoler MH, Williams BRG: Expression of the Wilms' tumor suppressor gene *WT1* during mouse embryogenesis. Cell Growth Differentiation 1993; 4:1023-1031.
3. Mundlos S, Pelletier J, Darveau A, Bachmann M, Winterpacht A, Zabel B: Nuclear localization of the protein encoded by the Wilms tumor gene WT1 in embryonic and adult tisuue. Develop 1993; 119:1329-1341.
4. Haber DA, Sohn RL, Buckler AJ, Pelletier J, Call KM, Housman DE: Alternative splicing and genomic structure of the Wilms tumor gene WT1. Proc Natl Acad Sci USA 1991; 88:9618-9622.
5. Mitchell PJ, Tjian R: Transcriptional regulation in mammalian cells by sequence-specific DNA binding proteins. Science 1989; 245:371-378.
6. Bray P, Lichter P, Thiesen HJ, Ward DC, Dawid IB: Characterization and mapping of human genes encoding zinc finger proteins. Proc Natl Acad Sci USA 1991; 88:9563-9567.
7. Huebner K, Druck T, Croce CM, Thiesen HJ: Twenty-seven nonoverlapping zinc finger cDNAs from human T cells map to nine different chromosomes with apparent clustering. Am J Hum Genet 1991; 48:726-740.

8. Stone B, Wharton W: Targeted RNA printing: the cloning of differentially-expressed cDNA fragments enriched for members of the zinc finger gene family. Nucl Acid Res 1994; 22:2612-2618.

9. Andreazzoli M, De Lucchini S, Costa M, Barsacchi G: RNA binding properties and evolutionary conservation of the Xenopus multifinger proetin Xfin. Nucl Acid Res 1993; 21:4218-4225.

10. Pabo CO, Sauer RT: Transcription factors: structural families and principles of DNA recognition. Annu Rev Bioch 1992; 61:1053-1095.

11. Pavletich NP, Pabo CO: Zinc finger-DNA recognition: crystal structure of a Zif268-DNA complex at 2.1 Å. Science 1991; 252:809-817.

12. Fairall L, Harrison SD, Travers AA, Rhodes D: Sequence-specific DNA binding by a two zinc-finger peptide from the Drosophila melanogaster Tramtrack Protein. J Mol Biol 1992; 226:349-366.

13. Thukral SK, Morrison ML, Young ET: Mutations in the zinc fingers of ADR1 that change the specificity of DNA binding and transactivation. Mol Cell Biol 1992; 12:2784-2792.

14. Nardelli J, Gibson T, Charnay P: Zinc finger-DNA recognition-Analysis of base specificity by site-directed mutagenesis. Nucl Acid Res 1992; 20:4137-4144.

15. Desjalais JR, Berg JM: Towards rules relating zinc finger protein sequences and DNA binding site preferences. Proc Natl Acad Sci USA 1992; 89:7345-7349.

16. Rauscher III F, Morris JE, Tournay OE, Cook DM, Curran T: Binding of the Wilms' tumor locus zinc finger protein to the EGR1 consensus sequence. Science 1990; 250:1259-1262.

17. Rangnekar VM, Aplin AC, Sukhatme VP: The serum and TPA responsive promoter and intron-exon structure of EGR2,a human early growth response gene encoding a zinc finger protein. Nucl Acid Res 1990; 18:2749-2757.

18. Sakamoto KM, Bardeleben C, Yates KE, Raines MA, Golde DW, Gasson JC: 5' Upstream sequence and genomic structure of the human primary response gene EGR-1/T1S8. Oncogene 1991; 6:867-871.

19. Patwardhan S, Gashler A, Siegel MG, Chang LC, Joseph LJ, Shows TB, Le BM, Sukhatme VP: EGR3, a novel member of the Egr family of genes encoding immediate-early transcription factors. Oncogene 1991; 6:917-928.

20. Holst C, Skerka C, Lichter P, Bilaonski A, Zipfel PF: Genomic organization, chromosomal localization and promotor function of the human zinc finger gene pAT133. Hum Mol Gent 1993; 2:367-372.

21. Ladanyi M, Gerald W: Fusion of the EWS and WT1 genes in the desmoplastic small round cell tumor. Cancer Res 1994; 54:2837-2840.

22. Kingsley C, Winoto A: Cloning of GT box-binding proteins: a novel Sp1 multigene family regulating T-cell receptor gene expression. Mol Cell Biol 1992; 12:4251-4261.

23. Harrington MA, Konicek B, Song A, Xia X, Fredericks WJ, Rauscher III FJ: Inhibition of colony-stimulating factor-1 promoter activity by the product of the Wilms tumor locus. J Biol Chem 1993; 268:21271-21275.

24. Bickmore WA, Oghene AK, Little MH, Seawright A, Van Heyningen V, Hastie ND: Modulation of DNA binding specificty by alternative splicing of the Wilms tumor WT1 gene transcript. Science 1992; 257:235-237.

25. Wang AQ, Qiu Q, Enger KT, Deuel TF: A second transcriptionally active DNA-binding site for the Wilms tumor gene product, WT1. Proc Natl Acad Sci USA 1993; 90:8896-8900.

26. Madden SL, Cook DM, Morris JF, Gashler A, Sukhatme VK, Rauscher III FJ: Transcriptional repression mediated by the WT1 tumor gene product. Science 1991; 253:1550-1553.

27. Drummond IA, Madden SL, Rohwer-Nutter P, Bell GI, Sukhatme VP, Rauscher III FJ: Repression of the insulin-like growth factor II gene by the Wilms tumor suppressor WT1. Science 1992; 257:674-678.

28. Gashler AL, Bonthron DT, Madden SL, Rauscher III FJ, Collins T, Sukhatme VP: Human platelet-derived growth factor A chain is transcriptionally repressed by the Wilms tumor suppressor WT1. Proc Natl Acad Sci USA 1992; 89:10984-10988.

29. Wang ZY, Madden SL, Deuel TF, Rauscher III FJ: The Wilms' tumor gene product, WT1, represses transcription of the platelet-derived growth factor A-chain gene. J Biol Chem 1992; 267:21999-22002.

30. Anant S, Axenovich SL, Madden SL, Rauscher III FJ, Subramanian KN: Novel replication inhibitory function of the developmental regulator/transcription repressor protein WT1 encoded by the Wilms tumor gene. Oncogene 1994; 9:3113-3126.

31. Hurwitz J, Adhya S, Field J, Gronostajski R, Guggenheimer RA, Kenny M, Lindenbaum J, Nagata N: Synthesis of adenoviral DNA with purified proteins. In Genetics, Cell Differentiation and Cancer. Academic Press, Inc., 1985.

32. Pruijn GJM, Van Driel W, Van der Vliet PC: Nuclear factor III, a novel sequence specific DNA binding protein from HeLa cells stimulating adenovirus replication. Nature 1986; 322:656-659.

33. Haber DA, Park S, Maheswaran S, Englert C, Re GG, Hazen-Martin DJ, Sens DA, Garvin AJ: WT-1-mediated growth suppression of Wilms tumor cells expressing WT1 splicing variant. Science 1993; 262:2057-2059.

34. Hastie ND: The genetics of Wilms' tumor. A case of dirupted development. Ann Review Genet 1994; 28:523-558.

35. Wang ZY, Qui QQ, Deuel TF: The Wilms tumor gene product WT1 activates or suppresses transcription through separate functional domains. J Biol Chem 1993; 268:9172-9175.

36. Werner H, Roberts Jr C, LeRoith D: The regulation of IGF-I receptor gene expression by positive and negative zinc-finger transcription factors. Adv Experiment Med Biol 1993; 343:91-103.

37. Werner HF, Rauscher III FJ, Sukhatme VP, Drummond IA, Roberts Jr C, LeRoith D: Transcriptional repression of the insulin-like growth factor I receptor (IGF-I-R) gene by the tumor suppressor WT1 involves binding to sequences both upstream and downstream of the IGF-I-R gene transcription start site. J Biol Chem 1994; 269:12577-12582.

38. Maheswaran S, Park S, Bernard A, Morris JF, Rauscher III FJ, Hill DE, Haber DA: Physical and functional interaction between WT1 and p53 proteins. Proc Natl Acad Sci USA 1993; 90: 5100-5104.

39. Madden SL, Cook DM, Rauscher III FJ: A structure-function analysis of transcriptional repression mediated by the WT1, Wilms tumor suppressor protein. Oncogene 1993; 8:1713-1720.

40. Werner H, Re GG, Drummond IA, Sukhatme VP, Rauscher III FJ, Sens DA, Garvin AJ, LeRoith D, Roberts Jr C: Increased expression of the insulin-like growth factor I receptor gene, IGFIR, in Wilms tumor is correlated with modulation of IGFIR promoter activity by the WT1 Wilms tumor gene product. Pro Natl Acad Sci USA 1993; 90:5828-5832.

41. Rupprecht HD, Drummond IA, Madden SL, Rauscher III FJ, Sukhatme VP: The Wilms tumor suppressor gene WT1 is negatively autoregulated. J Biol Chem 1994; 269:6198-6206.

42. Coppes MJ, Campbell CE, Williams BRG: The role of WT1 in Wilms tumorigenesis. FASEB J 1993; 7:886-895.

43. Drummond IA, Rupprecht HD, Rohwer-Nutter P, Lopez-Guisa JM, Madden SL, Rauscher III FJ, Sukhatme VP: DNA recognition by splicing variants of the Wilms tumor suppressor, WT1. Mol Cell Biol 1994; 14:3800-3809.

44. Haber DA, Buckler AJ, Glaser T, Call KM, Pelletier J, Sohn RL, Douglass EC, Housman DE: An internal deletion within an 11p13 zinc finger gene contributes to the development of Wilms' tumor. Cell 1990; 61:1257-1269.

45. Park S, Tomlinson G, Nisen P, Haber DA: Altered trans-activational properties of a mutated WT1 gene product in a WAGR-associated Wilm's tumor. Cancer Res 1993; 53:4757-4760.

46. Dey BR, Sukhatme VP, Roberts AB, Sporn MB, Rauscher III FJ, Kim SJ: Repression of the transforming growth factor-beta 1 gene by the Wilms tumor suppressor WT1 gene product. Molecular Endocrinology 1994; 8:595-602.

47. Reeve AE, Eccles MR, Wilkins RJ, Bell GI, Millow LJ: Expression of insulin-like growth factor-II transcripts in Wilms tumor. Nature 1985; 317:258-260.

48. Martinerie C, Huff V, Joubert I, Badzioch M, Saunders G, Strong L, Perbal B: Structural analysis of the human nov proto-oncogene and expression in Wilms tumor. Oncogene 1994; 9:2729-2732.

49. Haber DA, Timmers HT, Pelletier J, Sharp P, Housman DE: A dominant mutation in the Wilms tumor gene WT1 cooperates with the viral oncogene E1A in transformation of primary kidney cells. Proc Natl Acad Sci USA 1992; 89:6010-6014.

50. Sharma PM, Bowman M, Madden SL, Rauscher III FJ, Sukumar S: RNA editing in the Wilms tumor susceptibility gene, WT1. Genes Develop 1994; 8:720-731.

51. Teng B, Burant CF, Davidson NO: Molecular cloning of an apolipoprotein B messenger RNA editing protein. Science 1993; 260:1816-1818.

52. Hadjiagapiou C, Giannoni F, Funahashi SF, Davidson NO: Molecular cloning of a human small intestinal apolipoprotein B mRNA editing protein. Nucl Acid Res 1994; 22:1874-1879.

53. Morris JF, Madden SL, Tournay OE, Cook DM, Sukhatme VP, Rauscher III FJ: Characterization of the zinc finger protein encoded by the WT1 Wilms' tumor locus. Oncogene 1991; 6:2339-48.

54. Sharma PM, Bowman M, Yu B, Sukumar S: A rodent model for Wilms tumors: embryonal kidney neoplasms induced by N-nitroso-N'-methylurea. Proc Natl Acad Sci USA 1994; 91:9931-9935.

55. Roederer M, Staal FJ, Raju PA, Ela SW, Herzenberg LA, Herzenberg LA: Cytokine-stimulated human immunodeficiency virus replication is inhibited by N-acetyl-L-cysteine. Proc Natl Acad Sci USA 1990; 87:4884-4888.

56. Kalebic T, Kinter A, Poli G, Anderson ME, Meister A, Fauci AS: Suppression of human immunodeficiency virus expression in chronically infected monocytic cells by glutathione, glutathione ester, and N-acetylcysteine. Proc Natl Acad Sci USA 1991; 88:986-990.

57. Marui N, Offermann MK, Swerlick R, Kunsch C, Rosen CA, Ahmad M, Alexander RW, Medford RM: Vascular cell adhesion molecule-1 (VCAM-1) gene transcription and expression are regulated through an antioxidant-sensitive mechanism in human vascular endothelial cells. J Clin Invest 1993; 92:1866-1874.

58. Youngman LD, Park JY, Ames BN: Protein oxidation associated with aging is reduced by dietary restriction of protein or calories. Proc Natl Acad Sci USA 1992; 89:9112-9116.

59. Hockenbery DM, Oltvai ZN, Yin XM, Milliman CL, Korsmeyer SJ: Bcl-2 functions in an antioxidant pathway to prevent apoptosis. Cell 1993; 75:241-251.

60. Kane DJ, Sarafian TA, Anton R, Hahan H, Gralla EB, Valentine JS, Ord T, Bredesen DE: Bcl-2 inhibition of neural death: decreased generation of reactive oxygen species. Science 1993; 262:1274-1277.

61. Staal FJ, Roederer M, Herzenberg LA, Herzenberg LA: Intracellular thiols regulate activation of nuclear factor kappa B and transcription of human immunodeficiency virus. Proc Natl Acad Sci USA 1990; 87:9943-9947.

62. Schreck R, Rieber P, Baeuerle PA: Reactive oxygen intermediates as apparently widely used messengers in the activation of the NF-kappa B transcription factor and HIV-1. EMBO J 1991; 10: 2247-2258.

63. Matthews JR, Wakasugi N, Virelizier JL, Jodoi J, Hay RT: Thioredoxin regulates the DNA binding activity of NF-kappa B by reduction of a disulphide bond involving cysteine 62. Nucl Acid Res 1992; 20:3821-3830.

64. Storz G, Tartaglia A, Ames BA: Transcriptional regulator of oxidative stress-induced genes; direct activiation by oxidation. Science 1990; 248:189-194.

65. Tartaglia LA, Gimeno CJ, Storz G, Ames BN: Multidegenerate DNA recognition by the OxyR transcriptional regulator. J Biol Chem 1992; 267:2038-2045.

66. Toledano MB, Kullik I, Trinh F, Baird PT, Schneider TD, Storz G: Redox-dependent shift of OxyR-DNA contacts along an extended DNA-binding site: a mechanism for differential promoter selection. Cell 1994; 78:897-909.

67. Huang RP, Adamson ED: Characterization of the DNA-binding properties of the early growth response-1 (Egr-1) transcription factor: evidence for modulation by a redox mechanism. DNA Cell Biology 1993; 12:265-273.

68. Knoepfel L, Steinkuhler C, Carri MT, Rotilio G: Role of zinc-coordination and of the gluatathione redox couple in the redox susceptibility of human transcription factor Sp1. Biochem Biophys Res Comm 1994; 201:871-877.

69. Xanthoudakis S, Curran T: Identification and characterization of Ref-1, a nuclear protein that facilitates AP-1 DNA-binding activity. EMBO J 1992; 11:653-665.

70. Chandler D, el-Naggar AK, Brisbay S, Redline RW, McDonnell TJ: Apoptosis and expression of the bcl-1 proto-oncogene in the fetal and adult human kidney; evidence for the contribution of bcl-2 expression to renal carcinogenesis. Hum Pathol 1994; 25:789-796.

CHAPTER 7

NATURALLY OCCURRING MUTATIONS IN THE *WT1* GENE

INTRODUCTION

Dominant oncogenes, like *myc* or *ras*, confer a gain of function to transformed cells.[1,2] Gain-of-function mutations result in abnormal, positive signals for cell proliferation. In general, however, genetic alterations such as point mutations and deletions most often result in a loss of function and contribute to tumorigenesis by interference with mechanisms restraining cell proliferation. Such is the case for the Wilms tumor suppressor gene, *WT1*. Theoretically, mutations can occur at any site within the gene. However, it is important to consider whether the mutation results in the production of a modified protein (missense mutation) or in the production of a truncated WT1 protein (nonsense or frameshift mutation). Depending upon the biochemical function of the protein and the nature of its interaction with other proteins, missense or nonsense mutations could be expected to produce different phenotypes. And, indeed, constitutional missense mutations of the *WT1* gene appear to disrupt several organ systems and result in a far more severe phenotype (Denys-Drash syndrome — DDS, see chapter 1) than constitutional deletions (WAGR syndrome) or nonsense mutations (Wilms tumor only).

The first described 11p13 deletions in Wilms tumors encompassed more than one gene but, subsequently, intragenic mutations predicted to result in the functional inactivation of the WT1 protein were identified. Consequently, there now is strong evidence that the development of certain Wilms tumors conform to the two-hit

Wilms Tumor: Clinical and Molecular Characterization, by Max J. Coppes, Christine E. Campbell, and Bryan R.G. Williams. © 1995 R.G. Landes Company.

hypothesis, resulting from the inactivation of both alleles of the *WT1* gene. Moreover, it has been demonstrated that *WT1* germline mutations can result in a particular phenotype characterized by serious genitourinary malformations, nephropathy and Wilms tumor, i.e. DDS. Finally, *WT1* mutation analyses in tumors other than Wilms tumor suggest that *WT1* inactivation may play a role in the development of certain mesotheliomas.[3]

This chapter will review all *WT1* mutation analyses reported thus far in hereditary and non-hereditary Wilms tumors, in cancers other than Wilms tumor and in patients with the DDS.

WT1 MUTATIONS IN WILMS TUMOR

The first Wilms tumor to be analyzed in detail at a molecular level was Wit-13 (case #1, Table 7.1), a unilateral sporadic Wilms tumor carrying an estimated 175 kb homozygous deletion of a chromosome 11p13 region encompassing *WT1*.[4] However, the Wit-13 deletion is obviously relatively large and results in the inactivation of more than one gene. Similarly, a homozygous deletion in another tumor reported two years later was also large and encompassed more than one gene.[5] Subsequently, however, smaller deletions were reported. For example, a 16 *kB* homozygous deletion extending into *WT1* exon 1 (case #2, Table 7.1),[14] although, as it turns out, this deletion also inactivates *WIT1*, the gene co-localizing with *WT1* (see chapter 4). By contrast, the homozygous deletion extending 5' into *WT1* exon 10 described by Cowell et al (case #3, Table 7.1) does not extend telomerically as far as the adjacent 3' CpG island.[6] Since CpG islands are frequently associated with the 5' ends of expressed sequences, Cowell and colleagues claimed that their deletion does not affect any other known gene.[6]

The first homozygous intragenic mutations were reported in hereditary Wilms tumors. In 1991, Huff et al reported a 97 bp homozygous deletion in exon 6 of the *WT1* gene in both tumors of a one year old female (Table 7.1, #14) who had developed synchronous bilateral Wilms tumor.[11] This deletion shifts the reading frame of the mutant transcript, producing an in-frame termination codon, 22 nucleotides downstream of the deletion. As a result, the 180 carboxy-terminal amino acids present in the wild-type protein (containing the four zinc fingers) that constitute the DNA binding domain are predicted to be absent from the mutant protein. Of interest was the observation that the second event in

Table 7.1. Homozygous WT1 mutations in Wilms tumor specimens

No.	Patient/tumor (Ref)	WT1 mutation	Phenotype
1	WiT-13 [4]	175 kb deletion encompassing WT1	Sporadic unilateral Wilms tumor
2	ES [5]	16 kb deletion extending into WT1	Sporadic unilateral Wilms tumor
3	GOS 129 [6]	large deletion involving WT1 exon 10 only	Sporadic unilateral Wilms tumor
4	Wit-24 [7]	single nucleotide insertion (C) exon 10	Sporadic unilateral Wilms tumor
5	Wit-26 [7]	dinucleotide deletion (CpG) exon 10	Sporadic unilateral Wilms tumor
6	BT#53 [8]	C > T transition exon 8	Sporadic unilateral Wilms tumor
7	DJ#11 [8]	single nucleotide insertion (T) exon 9	Sporadic unilateral Wilms tumor
8	MF#88 [8]	deletion/insertion mutation exon 9	Sporadic unilateral Wilms tumor
9	BM#7 [8]	C > T transition exon 8 in one allele, 7 nucleotide insertion exon 3 in other allele	Sporadic unilateral Wilms tumor
10	Wit-29 [7,12]	C > T transition exon 8	De novo germline mutation, unilateral Wilms tumor
11	case 12 [9]	C > T transition exon 9	De novo germline mutation, unilateral Wilms tumor
12	GOS 543 [10]	constitutional 11p12-p13 deletion	Unilateral Wilms tumor in patient with WAGR
13	GOS 157 [10]	constitutional 11p12-p13 deletion	Unilateral Wilms tumor in patient with WAGR
		C > T transition exon 8	
14	209942 [11]	97 bp deletion exon 6	Bilateral Wilms tumor
15	PG [12]	17 bp deletion exon 4	Bilateral Wilms tumor, GU anomalies
16	NP57 [13]	C > T transition exon 9	Bilateral Wilms tumor (see NP58 Table 2)
17	TS [12]	single nucleotide deletion (G) exon 6	Familial Wilms tumor

each of the two tumors was different. The wild-type allele in the left Wilms tumor was lost due to a somatic recombination, while in the right tumor it was deleted due to chromosome loss and duplication. Since both tumors lost the maternal 11p allele during the second event, the 97 bp *WT1* exon 6 deletion (the 11p3 germline mutation) resided on the paternal chromosome. That same year, a second (17 bp *WT1* exon 4) intragenic germline deletion was reported in a patient with bilateral Wilms tumor and genitourinary malformations (Table 7.1, #15).[12] This frameshift mutation is expected to cause premature truncation of the protein, again eliminating the four zinc fingers.[12] These same investigators reported a second homozygous mutation, this time in a patient with Wilms tumor, whose father had also developed a Wilms tumor in childhood (Table 7.1, #17). The single nucleotide *WT1* deletion in exon 6 is also predicted to cause early termination of translation.[12] Of interest is the observation that the phenotypic expression of this constitutional mutation was more severe in the son, who was born with hypospadias and bilateral cryptorchidism in addition to his unilateral Wilms tumor (Table 7.1, #17), than in the father, who developed only Wilms tumor. Another example of a homozygous intragenic *WT1* mutation was provided in a patient with bilateral Wilms tumor.[13] The right-sided tumor of this patient carried a homozygous C to T transition in exon 9 of the *WT1* gene (Table 7.1, #16). This transition mutation converts an arginine residue, predicted to be involved in a guanine contact,[15] into a stop codon. However, the Wilms tumor in the left kidney of this same patient showed the same mutation in its heterozygous state (Table 7.2, #3).

Further analysis indicated that both tumors carried a T to G transversion in the intron between *WT1* exons 7 and 8.[13] However, the presence of the same intronic mutation in the unaffected father of this patient suggests that this alteration probably represents a polymorphism rather than a mutation.[13] Final examples of homozygous intragenic *WT1* mutation in hereditary Wilms tumor have been provided by two patients with unilateral sporadic Wilms tumor.[7,9] One patient was shown to carry a de novo germline mutation involving a C to T transition in *WT1* exon 8 (Table 7.1, #10), predicted to convert arginine to a premature stop codon,[7] the other carried a C > T transition in exon 9 (Table 7.1, #11), predicted to substitute tryptophane to arginine within the third

Table 7.2. Heterozygous WT1 mutations in Wilms tumor specimens

No.	Patient/tumor (Ref)	WT1 mutation	Phenotype
1	AR[16]	25 bp deletion spanning exon 9/intron region	Sporadic unilateral Wilms tumor
2	ZAGRE/WT10[13]	C > T transition exon 8	Sporadic unilateral Wilms tumor
3	NP58[13]	C > T transition exon 9	Bilateral Wilms tumor (see NP 57 Table 1)
4	AH#20[8]	deletion/insertion exon 8	Sporadic unilateral Wilms tumor
5	KK#33[8]	C > A transition exon 7	Sporadic unilateral Wilms tumor

zinc finger domain of WT1.[9] Interestingly, this mutation is identical to the most frequent point mutation associated with the DDS,[17] but this patient did not display the classical phenotypic triad associated with DDS.

In patients with the WAGR syndrome, the constitutional deletion involving chromosome 11p13 presumably represents the first hit and, if *WT1* is important in the development of these tumors, the remaining allele should also be mutant. The analysis of four tumors derived from three cases (one patient developed bilateral Wilms tumor) has revealed mixed results. In one unilateral Wilms tumor (Table 7.1, #12), the remaining allele was indeed shown to harbor a 10 bp insertion in exon 7 resulting in a frame shift and the generation of a stop codon.[18] Similarly, the unilateral Wilms tumor of a second WAGR patient (Table 7.1, #13) contained a C to T transition in exon 8 resulting in the immediate generation of a stop codon.[18] These two cases confirm the expectation that Wilms tumors in WAGR patients result from inactivation of *WT1*. However, no mutations were identified in either of the bilateral Wilms tumors in a third patient with WAGR, despite sequencing the complete *WT1* coding region. It remains possible that this patient carried a mutation outside the coding sequence, for example in the promotor region or in the 3' untranslated region.[19] Such mutations could modulate or affect transcript stability. Since expression of the *WT1* gene was not monitored in this case, the role of *WT1* remains speculative.

There are now several examples of homozygous somatic *WT1* inactivation in non-hereditary Wilms tumor. For instance, the homozygous C insertion in *WT1* exon 10 demonstrated in the tumor specimen of a four-year old boy who presented with unilateral Wilms tumor (Table 7.1, #4), as well as the homozygous CpG deletion in *WT1* exon 10 of a unilateral sporadic Wilms tumor of a two-year-old female (Table 7.1, #5).[7] Both mutations, which were absent in the constitutional cells, are predicted to disrupt the zinc finger motif.[15] In a recent analyses of 98 sporadic Wilms tumors, six additional patients with somatic *WT1* mutations were described (Table 7.1, # 6-9 and Table 7.2 # 4 and 5). Three of these (two *WT1* exon 9 mutations and one *WT1* exon 8 mutation) were found to be homozygous, two were heterozygous, while in one patient a different mutation was identified in each *WT1* allele (Table 7.1, #9). Both homozygous *WT1* exon 9 mutations (one a nonsense mutation and the other a deletion/insertion mutation, Table 7.1, #7 and #8) and the nonsense homozygous *WT1* exon 8 mutation (a C >T transition, Table 7.1, #6), are predicted to result in the production of a truncated WT1 protein.[8] The latter mutation (C >T transition in *WT1* exon 8) was also found heterozygously in another tumor (Table 7.1, #9). However, the second allele of that same tumor was shown to harbor a 7-nucleotide insertion in *WT1* exon 3, predicted to cause translational frameshifting. Consequently, this tumor specimen represents the first case of Wilms tumor with different mutations on both alleles predicted to result in the complete inactivation of *WT1*. The two remaining heterozygous mutations described by these investigators will be discussed in the next paragraphs.

Inactivation of *WT1* by a somatic point mutation followed by loss of the wild-type allele illustrates the classical two-hit mechanism for Wilms tumorigenesis. Most of the mutations reported thus far are confined to the zinc finger region (exons 7-10) of the *WT1* gene (Fig. 7.1). Mutations in *WT1* are clearly sufficient to initiate the development of certain Wilms tumor, but it remains to be determined what proportion of tumors actually involve homozygous mutations at this locus. Since approximately 20% of Wilms tumors manifest LOH for the region encompassing *WT1*,[20] a similar incidence of underlying *WT1* mutations might be expected. At this time, the number of cases reported with identified homozygous *WT1* mutations remains below expectation (5-10%).[7,8,13] Possible interpretations of this observation are discussed further in chapter 8.

In accord with the model that *WT1* mutations are generally recessive at the cellular level, most Wilms tumors are homozygous or hemizygous for the mutant allele. However, five Wilms tumors have been described in which the mutant *WT1* allele is present in a heterozygous state[8,13,16] (Table 7.2 and Fig. 7.2). These tumors could be accounted for by one or more of the following hypotheses. The apparently wild-type *WT1* allele may carry a mutation outside the coding region of the gene resulting in loss of expression at the protein level. Alternatively, the mutant form of the protein may interact with the wild-type form to interfere with its function in a dominant negative fashion, as has been proposed for *p53*.[21-23] A third possibility is that a combination of a single *WT1* mutation together with a mutation at a second locus may result in

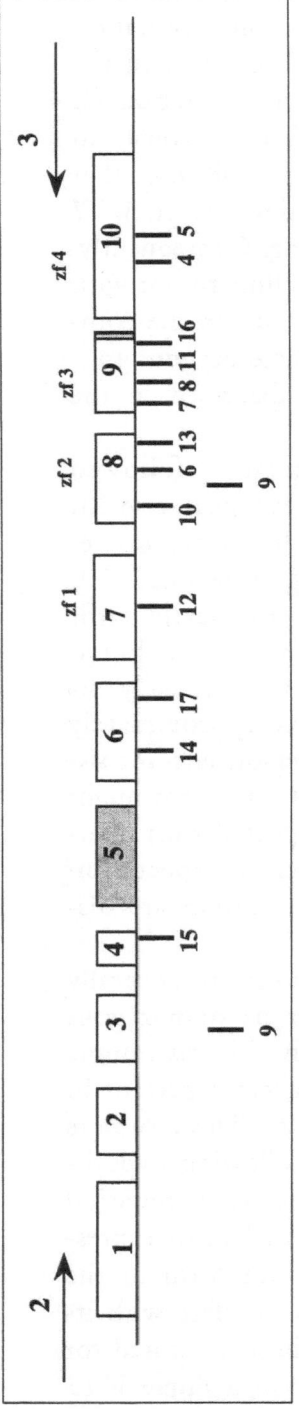

Fig. 7.1. Homozygous WT1 mutations in Wilms tumor. WT1 is encoded by 10 exons. A number of Wilms tumors have homozygous WT1 mutations (see also Table 7.1), including the following: (2) a deletion extending into exon 1,[14] (3) a deletion extending into exon 10,[6] (4) a single nucleotide insertion in exon 10,[7] (5) a dinucleotide deletion in exon 10,[7] (6) a C>T transition in exon 8,[8] (7) a single nucleotide insertion in exon 9,[8] (8) a deletion/insertion mutation in exon 9,[8] (9) a C>T transition in exon 8 in one allele and a 7 nucleotide insertion in exon 3 in the other allele,[8] (10) a C>T transition in exon 8,[7] (11) a C>T transition in exon 9,[9] (12) a 10 bp insertion in exon 7 in a patient with WAGR, i.e., with a constitutional 11p12-p13 deletion of the other allele,[18] (13) a C>T transition in exon 8 in a patient with WAGR, i.e., with a constitutional 11p12-p13 deletion of the other allele,[18] (14) a 97 bp deletion of exon 6,[11] (15) a 17 bp deletion in exon 4,[12] (16) a single nucleotide transition in exon 9 in one of the two tumors in a case with bilateral WT,[13] and (17) a single nucleotide deletion in exon 6.[12] Numbers under the bars in the figure and between brackets in bold in this legend correspond to patient numbers in Table 7.1.

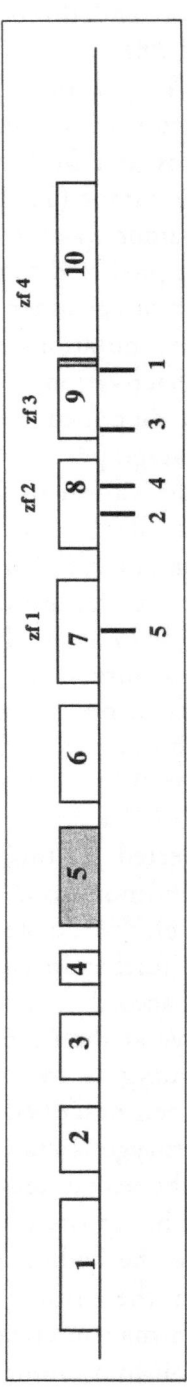

Fig. 7.2. Heterozygous WT1 mutations in Wilms tumor. A number of Wilms tumors have heterozygous WT1 mutations (see also Table 7.2), including the following: (1) a 25 bp deletion spanning the exon 9 /intron 9 junction,[16] (2) a C>T transition in exon 8,[13] (3) C>T transition in exon 9,[13] (4) a deletion/insertion in exon 8,[8] and (5) a C>A transition in exon 7.[8] Numbers under the bars in the figure and between brackets in bold in this legend correspond to patient numbers in Table 7.2.

a tumor phenotype. In support of this third hypothesis, Haber et al described a 25 bp heterozygous deletion spanning an exon-intron junction which lead to aberrant mRNA splicing and loss of the third zinc finger domain in the protein, in a unilateral Wilms tumor (Table 7.2, #1).[16] This tumor may only have expressed one mutated *WT1* gene either as a consequence of "trans-dominant suppression" or alternatively as the result of a second mutation within the untranslated *WT1* sequence affecting translation of the wild type transcript.[16] Although this tumor was heterozygous for *WT1*, chromosome 11 had undergone a nondisjunction event resulting in loss of one chromosome and duplication of the other. However, this event preceded the 25 bp deletion. It is possible that the early loss of one parental chromosome 11 was a random process, but it is also conceivable that this event rendered an earlier event elsewhere on chromosome 11 (11p15 for example) homozygous.[16] If this was the case, then more than one gene could be involved in the development of this particular Wilms tumor. This notion is not inconsistent with the two-hit hypothesis itself, since it predicts two rate-limiting steps but does not exclude additional genetic events that may be more frequent and may contribute to Wilms tumorigenesis. Additional support for Haber's hypothesis can be derived from observations of Henry and co-workers, who found that in two patients with the WAGR syndrome with a constitutional 11p13 deletion, tumor LOH was restricted to 11p15.[24] In these cases, the initial event would be the 11p13 lesion, transmitted in the germline, while the second somatic event is represented by chromosomal loss at 11p15.

Trans-dominant suppression was suggested as an explanation of additional heterozygous cases. A unilateral sporadic Wilms tumor (Table 7.2, #2) was shown to harbor a heterozygous C > T transition predicted to result in an arginine to cysteine change in zinc finger 2. In a second case, the tumor of the left kidney (NP 58) of a patient with synchronous bilateral Wilms tumor was demonstrated to be heterozygous for the constitutional C to T transition in exon 9 (Table 7.2, #3), while the right-sided tumor of this same patient (NP 57) was homozygous for this mutation (Table 7.1, #16). This nonsense mutation is predicted to convert an arginine residue into a stop codon. In both cases it is possible that there might have been other undetected changes in the remaining *WT1* allele, as only the sequence from the four zinc fingers was examined.[13] Cases #4 and #5 represent two additional examples of heterozygous somatic *WT1* mutations, one with a deletion/insertion in exon 8, predicted to result in a truncated *WT1* protein (Table 7.2, #4) and the other with a C > A transition in exon 7 (Table 7.2, #5). The latter missense mutation is predicted to convert [388]serine to tyrosine. Since this change occurs adjacent to a histidine residue involved in zinc chelation, Varanasi and co-workers suggested that this change might affect DNA binding.[8] The identification of *WT1* binding sites which can accommodate a function for the first *WT1* zinc finger in DNA recognition has confirmed this hypothesis (see chapter 6).

ANALYSIS OF *WT1* MUTATIONS IN TUMORS OTHER THAN WILMS TUMOR

The assumption that cells that normally express *WT1* constitute targets for pathological changes following its inactivation, led to the analysis of *WT1* mutations in tumors derived from tissues expressing *WT1*: granulosa cell (and other sex-cord stromal) tumors, mesotheliomas and endometrial cell carcinomas. In addition several other tumors have also been analyzed for *WT1* mutations.

GRANULOSA CELL TUMOR/SEX CORD-STROMAL TUMOR

Granulosa cell tumors are classified under the group of sex cord-stromal (SCS) tumors. SCS tumors are neoplasms of specialized gonadal stroma containing cells resembling Sertoli cells, Leydig cells, and granulosa cells, in varying combinations and degrees of differentiation. The observation that murine gonadal expression of *WT1* is restricted to the granulosa cells of the ovary and the Sertoli cells of the teses,[25] led to the evaluation of *WT1* in the development of tumors originating from these particular tissues.[26] Despite the fact that most granulosa cell tumors express *WT1*, no *WT1* zinc finger mutations were found in a small series of 11 cases.[26] Moreover, tumor LOH for two intragenic *WT1* polymorphic markers was excluded for 10 of the 11 specimens, suggesting that homozygous inactivation of *WT1* is not common in granulosa cell tumors.

MESOTHELIOMA

A detailed in situ hybridization analysis to identify the cell types responsible for *WT1* expression in adult mouse spleen, heart, lung and thymus, revealed that its expression is localized to the mesothelial cell lining of body cavities and the visceral organs such as heart, lung, intestine and liver.[3] In the spleen *WT1* expression is restricted to the supportive stromal cells and the splenic capsule. No detectable expression is seen in the splenocytes. Thus, *WT1* is only expressed in the connective structures of mesothelial origin. This observation led to the analysis of 32 asbestos-related mesotheliomas and one multicystic peritoneal mesothelioma, a proliferative lesion of borderline malignancy. Unlike the vast majority of mesotheliomas, the latter type of mesothelioma is not associated with a history of asbestos exposure. No *WT1* mutations were found in the 32 asbestos-related mesotheliomas.[3] However, the multicystic peritoneal mesothelioma contained a somatic homozygous A to G mutation in *WT1* exon 6, resulting in a serine to glycine substitution at codon 273.[3] Because insertion of this mutation into a *WT1* expression construct resulted in a protein that activated transcription from the EGR1 promotor, this mutation identifies a critical residue within the putative transactivation domain of *WT1* which is required for the transcriptional repression properties of this tumor suppressor protein.[3] Whether or not *WT1* plays an important role in other mesotheliomas still needs to be determined. The observation of malignant mesotheliomas arising in young adults who have been cured of Wilms tumor during their childhood[27] indicates the possibility that in certain cases germline mutations may confer a predisposition to both Wilms tumor and mesothelioma.

ENDOMETRIAL CARCINOMA

WT1 mRNA expression in endometrial cells as detected by in situ hybridization and immunohistochemistry studies of whole mount sections of Swiss Webster embryos was recently demonstrated.[28] No *WT1* expression was observed in the early stages of embryogenesis, however intense *WT1* expression was noted in the maternal uterus during this period of time.[28,29] No expression was observed in the epithelial lining of the gravid uterus, the trophoblastic cells, the ectoplacental cone of the embryoblast, or in the three germ cell layers of the embryo proper. During the phase of active organogenesis however, *WT1* expression was noted in the derivatives of the paramesonephric duct, the uterine body, uterine horn, and oviduct. Furthermore, certain endometrial carcinomas were shown to express *WT1*.[30] These results led to the study of the exonic sequence of the *WT1* zinc fingers in endometrial carcinoma.[30] The absence of *WT1* zinc finger mutations was confirmed by direct sequencing of biotinylated PCR products. It is of course possible that mutations might have occurred in areas of the *WT1* gene that were not covered or that in endometrial carcinomas, the function of the *WT1* gene might be altered as a result of posttranscriptional modifications or complexing with other intracellular factors leading to inactivation of the *WT1* gene product. Nevertheless, the results presented thus far suggest that *WT1* does not play a prominent role in the development of endometrial carcinomas, despite being expressed in some of these tumors.

OVARIAN CARCINOMA

Analysis of 40 cancers of the female reproductive tract, revealed that many ovarian carcinomas express *WT1* mRNA.[31] Northern blot analysis also indicated that in these tumors there were no gross rearrangements of the *WT1* gene leading to production of a mRNA species with altered mobility. Subsequent PCR-SSCP analysis failed to demonstrate mutations in any of the *WT1* exons. In conclusion, the significance of *WT1* mRNA expression in ovarian carcinoma is currently not understood, but the absence of *WT1* mutations suggests that *WT1* does not play an important role in its genesis.

TESTICULAR GERM CELL TUMOR

Testicular germ cell tumors (TGCTs) in adults show a consistent peritriploid DNA content with a relatively specific chromosomal distribution. Loss of parts or all of chromosomes 4, 5, 10, 11, 13 and 18 is common and LOH for chromosome 11p markers is observed in over 25% of cases.[32] The relatively high incidence of tumor specific LOH for markers at 11p15 and 11p13, led to the evaluation of 33 TGCTs (15 seminomas and 18 nonseminomatous germ cell tumors) primarily for mutations of the *WT1* zinc finger region,[32] despite the fact that germ cells are known not to express *WT1* mRNA. No aberrations were found in exons 2, 6 and 7-10,[32] nor were gross genomic changes of the *WT1* gene found using the cDNA probe WT33.[33] These data suggest that, while loss of genetic information from the short arm of chromosome 11 is relatively frequent, it does not seem to affect the *WT1* gene. Therefore, it seems unlikely that *WT1* plays a role in the development of these tumors.

CONSTITUTIONAL *WT1* MUTATIONS AND THE DENYS-DRASH SYNDROME

Occasionally Wilms tumor develops in individuals with intersex disorders, ambiguous genitalia and a characteristic nephropathy consisting of varying degrees of focal or diffuse mesangial sclerosis, a syndrome referred to as Denys-Drash syndrome (DDS) (see chapter 1). The notion that these three phenotypes of seemingly dissimilar disorders might have a common teratogenic origin affecting the kidney and the genital system has been confirmed at the molecular level. Huff et al,[34] and Pelletier et al,[35] were the first to describe constitutional *WT1* mutations in patients with DDS. Subsequently, additional reports have been published.[10,36-41] The mutations reported thus far are summarized in Table 7.3 and Figure 7.3.

The most common constitutional alteration found in DDS patients is a missense mutation that affects amino acid residue ^{394}Arg (a mutation in *WT1* exon 9, which encodes the third zinc finger). This mutation has been reported in 23 of 47 (≈50%) affected cases. The second most common constitutional alteration is a missense mutation that affect amino acid residue ^{396}Asp (exon 9 mutation). This mutation has been reported in 7/47 (~15%) cases. Other less common missense mutations affect amino acid residue ^{377}His (exon 8), ^{373}His (exon 8), ^{366}Arg (exon 8), ^{360}Cys (exon 8), ^{355}Cys (exon 8), and ^{330}Cys (exon 7). Also, three frameshift mutations have been reported, starting at amino acid ^{387}Thr (exon 9), ^{362}Arg (exon 8), and ^{275}Asn (exon 6) respectively. In addition, intron 9 mutations, which prevent splicing at one of the alternative splice donor sites of exon 9, have been reported in three DDS patients. An 11p12-13 deletion was demonstrated in another patient with DDS, while there have also been two cases reported with no mutations in the coding sequence of *WT1*,[10,41] although an intron 9 mutation was not excluded in either case. While mutations affecting different *WT1* exons can give rise to DDS, exon 9 seems to be a "hot spot" for constitutional mutations causing the DDS (see Fig. 7.3).

The demonstration that single constitutional *WT1* point mutations in DDS have more severe effects than the large constitutional deletions, demonstrated in several WAGR patients or in the

Table 7.3. Constitutional mutations in patients with the Denys-Drash syndrome

No.	Patient ref	Karyotype	Exon	Mutation	External Genitalia	Internal Genitalia	Nephropathy	Tumor
1	D1 [37]	46,XX	9	394Arg to Trp	Female	Normal ovaries/uterus	+	Bilateral Wilms tumor
2	D5 [37]	46,XY	9	394Arg to Trp	Ambiguous	normal testes, residual Müllerian structures	+	Prophylactic nephrectomies
3	AM [35]	ND	9	394Arg to Trp	Ambiguous	ND	+	-
4	CB [35]	46,XY	9	394Arg to Trp	Ambiguous	Dysgenic testes, bilateral Müllerian but no Wolffian structures	+	Bilateral gonadoblastoma, Wilms tumor
5	AU [35]	46,XX	9	394Arg to Trp	Female	ND	+	Bilateral Wilms tumor
6	PJ [35]	46,XY	9	394Arg to Trp	Ambiguous	Dysgenic R testis, normal L testis bicomal uterus	+	Unilateral Wilms tumor
7	SE [35]	46,XX	9	394Arg to Trp	Female	Normal	+	Unilateral Wilms tumor
8	MW [35]	46,XX	9	394Arg to Trp	Female	Dysgenic R gonad, L streak gonad normal uterus and vagina	+	Unilateral Wilms tumor
9	RS [35]	46, XY	9	394Arg to Trp	Ambiguous	Dysgenic testes	+	Unilateral Wilms tumor
10	LW [36]	46,XY	9	394Arg to Trp	Ambiguous	Rudimentary uterus	+	Wilms tumor
11	MA [10]	46,XY	9	394Arg to Trp	Ambiguous	Not specified genital anomalies	+	Unilateral Wilms tumor
12	HD [10]	46,XY	9	394Arg to Trp	Female	Not specified genital anomalies	+	Prophylactic nephrectomies
13	LB [10, 39]	46,XY	9	394Arg to Trp	Female	Female	+	Unilateral Wilms tumor
14	TG [17]	46,XY	9	394Arg to Trp	Ambiguous	ND	+	-
15	J [17]	46,XY	9	394Arg to Trp	ND	ND	+	Wilms tumor
16	IV [17]	ND	9	394Arg to Trp	ND	ND	+	Wilms tumor
17	802646 [17]	ND	9	394Arg to Trp	ND	ND	+	-
18	802669 [17]	ND	9	394Arg to Trp	ND	ND	+	Unknown
19	85-583 [40]	46,XY	9	394Arg to Trp	Female	ND	+	-
20	D3 [41]	46,XY	9	394Arg to Trp	ND	Hypospadias, bifid scrotum bilateral cryptorchidism	+	Nephrectomy, no tumor found
21	1560 [42]	46,XX	9	394Arg to Trp	Female	Apparently normal	+	Unilateral Wilms tumor
22	1658 [42]	46,XY	9	394Arg to Trp	Female	Dysgenic gonads	+	-
23	JK [36]	46,XY	9	394Arg to Pro	Female	ND	+	Wilms tumor
24	WY [35]	46,XY	9	396Asp to Asn	Ambiguous	L Wolffian structure, no Müllerian structures	+	Unilateral Wilms tumor

Patient	Identifier	Karyotype	Exon	Mutation	Phenotypic sex	Gonads/genitalia		Tumor/outcome
25	SS[10]	46,XY	9	396Asp to Asn	Male	normal	+	Bilateral Wilms tumor
26	802629[17]	46,XY	9	396Asp to Asn	Ambiguous	ND	+	-
27	D2[41]	46,XY	9	396Asp to Asn	ND	Hypospadias, bifid scrotum bilateral cryptorchidism	+	Wilms tumor
28	D5[41]	46,XX	9	396Asp to Asn	Female	No anomalies	+	Wilms tumor
29	2[43]	46,XX	9	396Asp to Asn	Female	ND	+	Bilateral Wilms tumor
30	BE[35]	46,XX	9	396Asp to Gly	Female	ND	+	-
31	[38]	46,XY	9	387Thr-frameshift	Male	hypospadias, bilateral undescended testes	+	-
32	CS[36]	46,XY	intron 9		Female	Streak gonads, infantile uterus	+	Wilms tumor
33	II[17]	ND	intron 9		ND	ND	+	Wilms tumor
34	III[17]	ND	intron 9		ND	ND	+	Wilms tumor
35	1614[42]	46,XX	8	355Cys to Tyr	Female	Apparently normal	+	Unilateral Wilms tumor
36	R7[39]	46,XY	8	360Cys to Tyr	Female	Infantile testes, no Müllerian structures	+	Died at age 6 1/2 months No tumor
37	3[43]	ND	8	360Cys to Gly	Female	Micropenis, cryptorchidism	+	Unilateral Wilms tumor
38	4[43] S12[39]	46,XY	8	362Arg-frameshift	ND	Dysgenic R testes, L streak gonad no Müllerian/Wolffian structures	+	Bilateral Wilms tumor
39	SV[35]	46,XY	8	366Arg to His	Female		+	Gonadoblastoma
40	LVH[10]	46,XY	8	366Arg to His	Ambiguous	ND	+	Unilateral Wilms tumor
41	WT5100[17]	46,XY	8	373His to Gln	Female	Partially bicornuate uterus R gonadal streak	+	Bilateral Wilms tumor L Gonadoblastoma
42	5[43]	46,XY	8	373His to Gln	ND	Hypospadias	+	Unilateral Wilms tumor
43	D10[40]	46,XY	8	377His to Tyr	Female	Streak gonads	+	Prophylactic nephrectomies
44	D1[41]	46,XY	8	377His to Arg	ND	Hypospadias, bifid scrotum	+	Wilms tumor
45	KJ[36]	46,XX	7	330Cys to Tyr	ND	ND	+	-
46	PM[10]	46,XY	6	275Asn-frameshift	Ambiguous	Atrophic gonads	+	Bilateral Wilms tumor
47	PD[10]	46,XX	11p12-13 del		Female	Normal	+	Unilateral Wilms tumor

The molecular analyses of virtually all patients presented was performed on constitutional DNA from the patients. ND= not determined; R= right; L= left; Patient #4 also developed a juvenile granulosa cell tumor; patient #37 also had cerebral atrophy and psychomotor delay; patient #38 has gross motor delay, craniostenosis and a horseshoe kidney; patient #47 has mental retardation and aniridia.

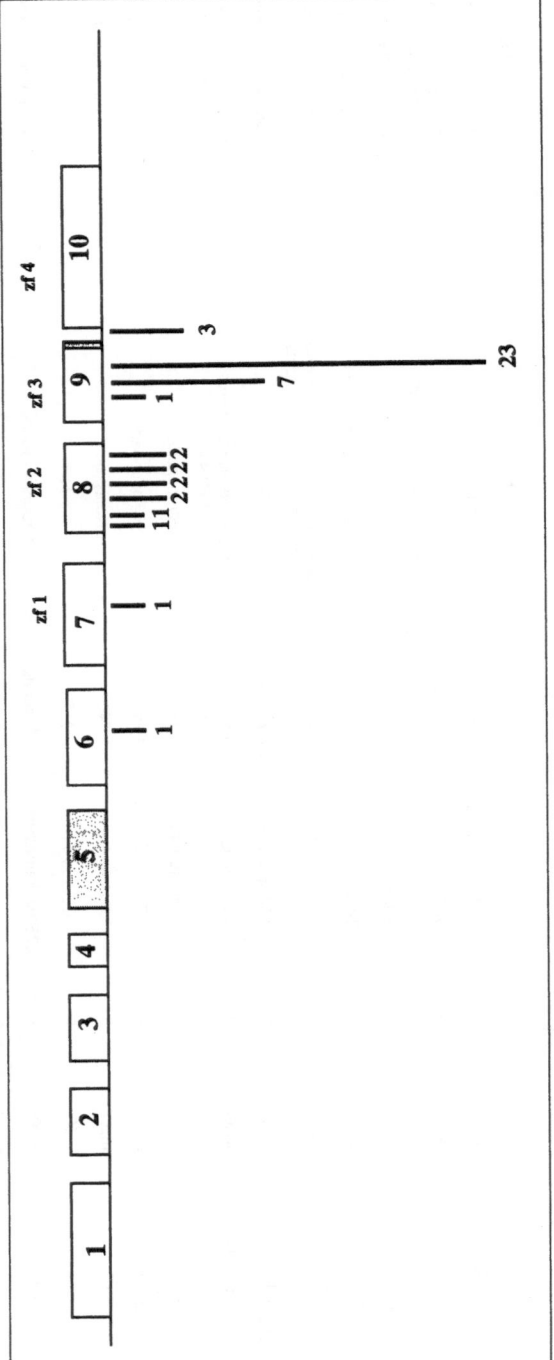

Fig. 7.3. Constitutional mutations in patients with Denys-Drash syndrome. Mutations in DDS have been reported for 46/49 patients analyzed. One patient (Table 7.2, #47) has an 11p12-13 deletion, while in two additional patients no mutation was detected in the coding region of WT1. The remaining 46 patients harbor single nucleotide changes. The bars indicate the position of the DDS mutations. The number underneath the bar designates the number of patients with DDS who harbor that particular mutation. For details on the mutations see Table 7.2.

QUESTIONNAIRE

Receive a FREE BOOK of your choice

Please help us out—Just answer the questions below, then select the book of your choice from the list on the back and return this card.

R.G. Landes Company publishes five book series: *Medical Intelligence Unit, Molecular Biology Intelligence Unit, Neuroscience Intelligence Unit, Tissue Engineering Intelligence Unit* and *Biotechnology Intelligence Unit*. We also publish comprehensive, shorter than book-length reports on well-circumscribed topics in molecular biology and medicine. The authors of our books and reports are acknowledged leaders in their fields and the topics are unique. Almost without exception, there are no other comprehensive publications on these topics.

Our goal is to publish material in important and rapidly changing areas of bioscience for sophisticated scientists. To achieve this goal, we have accelerated our publishing program to conform to the fast pace in which information grows in bioscience. Most of our books and reports are published within 90 to 120 days of receipt of the manuscript.

Please circle your response to the questions below.

1. We would like to sell our *books* to scientists and students at a deep discount. But we can only do this as part of a prepaid subscription program. The retail price range for our books is $59-$99. Would you pay $196 to select four *books* per year from any of our Intelligence Units–$49 per book–as part of a prepaid program?

           Yes   No

2. We would like to sell our *reports* to scientists and students at a deep discount. But we can only do this as part of a prepaid subscription program. The retail price range for our reports is $39-$59. Would you pay $145 to select five *reports* per year–$29 per report–as part of a prepaid program?

           Yes   No

3. Would you pay $39–the retail price range of our books is $59-$99–to receive any single book in our Intelligence Units if it is spiral bound, but in every other way identical to the more expensive hardcover version?

           Yes   No

To receive your free book, please fill out the shipping information below, select your free book choice from the list on the back of this survey and mail this card to:

    R.G. Landes Company, 909 S. Pine Street, Georgetown, Texas 78626 U.S.A.

Your Name _____

Address _____

City_____ State/Province:_____

Country: _____ Postal Code:_____

My computer type is Macintosh_____ ; IBM-compatible _____ ; Other _____

Do you own ____ or plan to purchase ___ a CD-ROM drive?

AVAILABLE FREE TITLES

Please check three titles in order of preference.
Your request will be filled based on availability. Thank you.

☐ Water Channels
Alan Verkman,
University of California-San Francisco

☐ The Na,K-ATPase:
Structure-Function Relationship
J.-D. Horisberger, University of Lausanne

☐ Intrathymic Development of T Cells
J. Nikolic-Zugic,
Memorial Sloan-Kettering Cancer Center

☐ Cyclic GMP
Thomas Lincoln, University of Alabama

☐ Primordial VRM System and the Evolution
of Vertebrate Immunity
John Stewart, Institut Pasteur-Paris

☐ Thyroid Hormone Regulation
of Gene Expression
Graham R. Williams, University of Birmingham

☐ Mechanisms of Immunological Self Tolerance
Guido Kroemer, CNRS Génétique Moléculaire et
Biologie du Développement-Villejuif

☐ The Costimulatory Pathway
for T Cell Responses
Yang Liu, New York University

☐ Molecular Genetics of Drosophila Oogenesis
Paul F. Lasko, McGill University

☐ Mechanism of Steroid Hormone Regulation
of Gene Transcription
M.-J. Tsai & Bert W. O'Malley, Baylor University

☐ Liver Gene Expression
François Tronche & Moshe Yaniv,
Institut Pasteur-Paris

☐ RNA Polymerase III Transcription
R.J. White, University of Cambridge

☐ src Family of Tyrosine Kinases in Leukocytes
Tomas Mustelin, La Jolla Institute

☐ MHC Antigens and NK Cells
Rafael Solana & Jose Peña,
University of Córdoba

☐ Kinetic Modeling of Gene Expression
James L. Hargrove, University of Georgia

☐ PCR and the Analysis of the T Cell Receptor
Repertoire
Jorge Oksenberg, Michael Panzara & Lawrence
Steinman, Stanford University

☐ Myointimal Hyperplasia
Philip Dobrin, Loyola University

☐ Transgenic Mice as an In Vivo Model
of Self-Reactivity
David Ferrick & Lisa DiMolfetto-Landon,
University of California-Davis and Pamela Ohashi,
Ontario Cancer Institute

☐ Cytogenetics of Bone and Soft Tissue Tumors
Avery A. Sandberg, Genetrix & Julia A. Bridge ,
University of Nebraska

☐ The Th1-Th2 Paradigm and Transplantation
Robin Lowry, Emory University

☐ Phagocyte Production and Function Following
Thermal Injury
Verlyn Peterson & Daniel R. Ambruso,
University of Colorado

☐ Human T Lymphocyte Activation Deficiencies
José Regueiro, Carlos Rodríguez-Gallego
and Antonio Arnaiz-Villena,
Hospital 12 de Octubre-Madrid

☐ Monoclonal Antibody in Detection and
Treatment of Colon Cancer
Edward W. Martin, Jr., Ohio State University

☐ Enteric Physiology of the Transplanted Intestine
Michael Sarr & Nadey S. Hakim, Mayo Clinic

☐ Artificial Chordae in Mitral Valve Surgery
Claudio Zussa, S. Maria dei Battuti Hospital-Treviso

☐ Injury and Tumor Implantation
Satya Murthy & Edward Scanlon,
Northwestern University

☐ Support of the Acutely Failing Liver
A.A. Demetriou, Cedars-Sinai

☐ Reactive Metabolites of Oxygen and Nitrogen
in Biology and Medicine
Matthew Grisham, Louisiana State-Shreveport

☐ Biology of Lung Cancer
Adi Gazdar & Paul Carbone,
Southwestern Medical Center

☐ Quantitative Measurement
of Venous Incompetence
Paul S. van Bemmelen, Southern Illinois University
and John J. Bergan, Scripps Memorial Hospital

☐ Adhesion Molecules in Organ Transplants
Gustav Steinhoff, University of Kiel

☐ Purging in Bone Marrow Transplantation
Subhash C. Gulati,
Memorial Sloan-Kettering Cancer Center

☐ Trauma 2000: Strategies for the New Millennium
David J. Dries & Richard L. Gamelli,
Loyola University

patients with large homozygous deletions encompassing the *WT1* gene, is intriguing and indicates that the mutations in patients with the DDS must result in more than simply inactivation or reduction of *WT1* gene expression. This suggests that the presence of a dysfunctional WT1 protein results in a more severe phenotype than complete inactivation or absence of the same protein. This may be explained by the "dominant negative" mechanism.[43]

What evidence do we have that certain constitutional *WT1* mutations cause the three phenotype that constitute the DDS? Our current knowledge seems to support a role for *WT1* in the development of each of the three features. A role for *WT1* in the development of Wilms tumor is clear from the evidence summarized above. In cases analyzed, the constitutional *WT1* mutations associated with DDS have been found to be reduced to homozygosity in the Wilms tumors isolated from these individuals. Proof of a role in the development of the renal mesangial sclerosis described in all DDS cases, has yet to be established. However, it is reasonable to hypothesize that disturbances of the WT1 protein result in aberrant differentiation and hypertrophy of the glomerular epithelium of the developing kidney, the precursor cells involved in the aberrant structures demonstrated in the kidneys of patients with the DDS.[35] These cells express high levels of the *WT1* mRNA in human embryonic kidneys as revealed by in situ hybridization.[44] Consequently, the renal failure seen in most DDS patients should be considered as a secondary phenomenon to the pathologic glomerular development. Finally, there are several reports suggesting that germline mutations in *WT1* are responsible for the development of certain genitourinary malformations, such as the ones described in DDS. Indirect evidence is provided by the demonstration of *WT1* expression in the genital ridge and fetal gonads of the human[44] and murine embryos.[25] In addition, constitutional *WT1* mutations have been demonstrated in patients with Wilms tumor who also presented with serious genitourinary malformations, but did not have all three criteria of DDS.[12] Together, these data support a role for *WT1* in the etiology of all three phenotypes of the DDS.

Not all individuals with constitutional *WT1* mutations exhibit all characteristics of DDS. The patient with synchronous bilateral Wilms tumor reported by Little et al (Table 7.1, #7 and 13) with a constitutional C to T point mutation in *WT1* exon 9 predicted to result in early termination of translation had neither genitourinary malformations nor nephropathy.[13] Both patients PG (Table 7.1, #5) and TS (Table 7.1, #6) had genitourinary malformations, but no intersex disorders or nephropathy.[12] Also, patient Wit-29 (Table 7.1, #8)), only presented with a sporadic unilateral Wilms tumor and no other phenotypes.[7] Finally, one phenotypically normal individual has been reported with a constitutional *WT1* mutation. This individual is the father of DDS patient D5 (Table 7.1, #2). Both father and son carry the same *WT1* exon 9 mutation (the one described in 20 of 36 DDS cases), but only the son is phenotypically affected.[37] These data imply that, while in almost all DDS patients, constitutional *WT1* mutations have been described, not all constitutional *WT1* mutations result in DDS.[7,9] Possible explanations for these rare individuals include the existence of non-allelic suppressor mutations or alternatively one could hypothesize that in some individuals the mutant *WT1* allele is not expressed during the crucial developmental stages. It should be kept in mind that, since the WT1 protein has not been studied in many Wilms tumors or in any patients with DDS, it remains possible that some of the mutant alleles are not expressed.

It is interesting to note that virtually all of the *WT1* mutations described to date are predicted to alter the DNA binding affinity of the gene product. The majority of mutations described in Wilms tumors are recessive nonsense or frame shift mutations (Table 7.1 and 7.2, Figs. 7.1 and 7.2), while the majority of mutations described in DDS are dominant missense mutations (Table 7.3, Fig. 7.3). Most of these missense mutations affect amino acids which have been shown in other zinc finger proteins to be involved in coordinating the zinc ion or in making contacts with the DNA[15] (see chapter 6). The most common DDS mutation, ^{394}Arg -^{394}Trp, is especially interesting in this regard as it alters an amino acid probably involved in sequence binding specificity, raising the possibility that this particular mutant WT1 protein might exert its influence on phenotype as a result of binding to inappropriate DNA sequences. The DDS alterations are primarily missense mutations in the second and third zinc fingers, although a single missense mutation affecting zinc finger 1 has been described as well as a nonsense mutation in exon 6. No missense mutations have been described to date in the putative transactivation domain of *WT1* in DDS.

It is also noteworthy that most single nucleotide mutations in *WT1* occur at an arginine residue. Transitions at CpG dinucleotides also contribute heavily to the *p53* mutation frequency in many cancers, although the fraction of tumor mutations that are transitions at CpG sites varies greatly from one cancer type to another. Moreover, over one-third of all point mutations giving rise to human genetic disease are due to mutation from CpG to TpG, despite the rarity of CpGs and the existence of a dedicated repair system. The unusual mutability of CpG dinucleotides is attributed to the presence of 5-methylcystine residues found at these dinucleotide sites.

CONCLUSION

Current evidence shows that *WT1* plays a role in the initiation of Wilms tumor. However, since *WT1* gene mutations have been demonstrated only in a limited number of cases (~5%), *WT1* is likely involved in only a subset of Wilms tumors. This is perhaps not surprising given the genetic evidence for the involvement of other loci that has accumulated in the past few years. Moreover, the 11p13 locus itself is complex. A second gene *WIT1*, which is closely linked to *WT1*, is coordinately expressed with *WT1* in embryonic kidney and most Wilms tumors, suggesting that both transcripts are co-regulated or may be transcriptionally-interdependent. Thus, tumor LOH for chromosome 11p13 markers presently estimated at 20% could unmask mutations exclusively localized to *WIT1*. Alternatively, mutations could occur in the promotor region of *WT1/WIT1*. Only further molecular analyses will resolve this issue.

The observation of constitutional *WT1* mutations in virtually all patients with DDS provides a molecular basis for this syndrome, although there are exceptions where constitutional *WT1* mutations do not exhibit all or any of the three phenotypes characteristic of DDS. Whether constitutional *WT1* mutations are involved in intersex or renal disorders not associated with DDS remains to be established.

Finally, it will be interesting to learn whether tumors other than Wilms tumor can develop as a consequence of *WT1* inactivation. Preliminary data suggest that not many tumors will, although the data presented thus far has been limited both in the number of tumors analyzed and in the *WT1* region screened (mostly the zinc finger region). However, based on its restricted pattern of expression, it seems unlikely that many different tumors will develop as a consequence of the inactivation of the *WT1* gene.

REFERENCES

1. Marcu KB, Bossone SA, Patel AJ: myc functiuon and regulation. Ann Rev Biochem 1992; 61:809-860.

2. Lowy DR, Willumsen BM: Function and regaulation of ras. Ann Rev Biochem 1992; 62:851-891.

3. Park S, Schalling M, Bernard A, Maheswaran S, Shipley GC, Roberts D, Fletcher J, Shipman R, Rheinwald J, Demetri G, Griffin J, Minden M, Housman DE, Haber DA: The Wilms tumour gene WT1 is expressed in murine mesoderm-derived tissues and mutated in a human mesothelioma. Nature Genetics 1993; 4:415-420.

4. Lewis WH, Yeger H, Bonetta L, Chan HLS, Kang J, Junien C, Cowell J, Jones C, Dafoe LA: Homozygous deletion of a DNA marker from chromosome 11p13 in sporadic Wilms tumor. Genomics 1988; 3:25-31.

5. Gessler M, Poustka A, Cavenee W, Neve RL, Orkin SH, Bruns GA: Homozygous deletion in Wilms tumours of a zinc-finger gene identified by chromosome jumping. Nature 1990; 343:774-778.

6. Cowell JK, Wadey RB, Haber DA, Call KM, Housman DE, Pritchard J: Structural rearrangements of the WT1 gene in Wilms' tumour cells. Oncogene 1991; 6:595-599.

7. Coppes MJ, Liefers GJ, Paul P, Yeger H, Williams BRG: Homozygous somatic *WT1* point mutations in sporadic unilateral Wilms tumor. Proc Natl Acad Sci USA 1993; 90:1416-1419.

8. Varanasi R, Bardeesy N, Ghahremani M, Petruzzi M-J, Nowak N, Adam MA, Grundy P, Shows TB, Pelletier J: Fine structure analysis of the *WT1* gene in sporadic Wilms tumors. Proc Natl Acad Sci USA 1994; 91:3554-3558.

9. Akasaka Y, Kikuchi H, Nagai T, Hiraoka N, Kato S, Hata J: A point mutation found in the WT1 gene in a sporadic Wilms' tumor without genitourinary abnormalities is identical with the most frequent point mutation in Denys-Drash syndrome. FEBS 1993; 317:39-43.

10. Baird PN, Santos A, Groves N, Jadresic L, Cowell JK: Constitutional mutations in the WT1 gene in patients with Denys-Drash syndrome. Hum Molec Genet 1992; 1:301-305.

11. Huff V, Miwa H, Haber DA, Call KM, D. H, Strong LC, G.F. S: Evidence for WT1 as a Wilms' tumor (WT) gene: intragenic germinal deletion in bilateral WT. Am J Hum Genet 1991; 48:997-1003.

12. Pelletier J, Bruening W, Li FP, Haber DA, Glaser T, Housman DE: WT1 mutations contribute to abnormal genital system development and hereditary Wilms' tumour. Nature 1991; 353:431-434.

13. Little MH, Prosser J, Condie A, Smith PJ, Van Heyningen V, Hastie ND: Zinc finger point mutations within the WT1 gene in Wilms tumor patients. Proc Natl Acad Sci USA 1992; 89: 4791-4795.

14. Ton CC, Huff V, Call KM, Cohn S, Strong LC, Housman DE, Saunders GF: Smallest region of overlap in Wilms tumor deletions uniquely implicates an 11p13 zinc finger gene as the disease locus. Genomics 1991; 10:293-297.

15. Pavletich NP, Pabo CO: Zinc finger-DNA recognition: crystal structure of a Zif268-DNA complex at 2.1 Å. Science 1991; 252: 809-817.

16. Haber DA, Buckler AJ, Glaser T, Call KM, Pelletier J, Sohn RL, Douglass EC, Housman DE: An internal deletion within an 11p13 zinc finger gene contributes to the development of Wilms' tumor. Cell 1990; 61:1257-1269.

17. Coppes MJ, Campbell CE, Williams BRG: The role of *WT1* in Wilms tumorigenesis. FASEB 1993; J 7:886-895.

18. Baird PN, Groves N, Haber DA, Housman DE, Cowell JK: Identification of mutations in the WT1 gene tumours from patients with the WAGR syndrome. Oncogene 1992; 7:2141-2149.

19. Fraizier GC, Wu Y-J, Hewitt SM, Maity T, Ton CCT, Huff V, Saunders GF: Transcriptional regulation of the human Wilms tumor gene (WT1). J Biol Chem 1994; 269:8892-8900.

20. Coppes MJ, Bonetta L, Huang A, Hoban P, Chilton-MacNeill S, Campbell CE, Weksberg R, Yeger H, Reeve AE, Williams BRG: Loss of heterozygosity mapping in Wilms tumor indicates the involvement of three distinct regions and a limited role for non-disjunction or mitotic recombination. Genes Chrom Cancer 1992; 5:326-334.

21. Herskowitz I: Functional inactivation of genes by dominant negative mutations. Nature 1987; 329:219-222.

22. Finlay CA, Hinds PW, Levine AJ: The p53 proto-oncogene can act as a suppressor of transformation. Cell 1989; 57:1083-1093.

23. Lavigueur A, Maltby V, Mock D, Rossant J, Pawson T, Bernstein A: High incidence of lung, bone, and lymphoid tumors in transgenic mice overexpressing mutant alleles of the p53 oncogene. Mol Cell Biol 1989; 9:3982-3991.

24. Henry I, Grandjouan S, Couillin P, Barichard F, Huerre-Jeanpierre C, Glaser T, Philip T, Lenoir G, Chaussain JL, Junien C: Tumor-specific loss of 11p15.5 alleles in del11p13 Wilms tumor and in familial adrenocortical carcinoma. Proc Natl Acad Sci USA 1989; 86:3247-3251.

25. Pelletier J, Schalling M, Buckler AJ, Rogers A, Haber DA, Housman D: Expression of the Wilms' tumor gene WT1 in the murine urogenital system. Genes Dev 1991; 5:1345-1356.

26. Coppes MJ, Ye Y, Rackley R, Zhao X-l, Liefers GJ, Casey G, Williams BRG: Analysis of *WT1* in granulosa cell and other sex cord-stromal tumors. Cancer Res 1993; 53:2712-2714.

27. Austin MB, Fechner RE, Roggli VL: Pleural malignant mesothelioma following Wilms' tumor. Am J Clin Pathol 1986;
86:227-230.

28. Rackley RR, Flenniken AM, Kuriyan NP, Kessler PM, Stoler MH,
Williams BRG: Expression of the Wilms' tumor suppressor gene
WT1 during mouse embryogenesis. Cell Growth Differentiation
1993; 4:1023-1031.

29. Zhou J, Rauscher FJ III, Bondy C: Wilms' tumor (WT1) gene
expression in decidual differentiation. Differentiation 1993;
54:109-114.

30. Rackley R, Casey G, Zhao X-l, Miller DW, Williams BRG, Coppes
MJ: Analysis of the Wilms tumor suppressor gene *WT1* in endometrial carcinoma. Genes Chrom Cancer 1994.

31. Bruening W, Gros P, Sato T, Stanirmir J, Nakamura Y, Housman
D, Pelletier J: Analysis of the 11p13 Wilms' tumor suppressor gene
(WT1) in ovarian tumors. Cancer Investigat 1993; 11:393-399.

32. Looijenga LHJ, Abraham M, Gillis AJM, Saunders GF, Oosterhuis
JW: Testicular germ cell tumors of adults show deletions of chromosomal bands 11p13 and 11p15.5, but no abnormalities within
the zinc-finger regions and exons 2 and 6 of the Wilms' tumor I
gene. Genes Chrom Cancer 1994; 9:153-160.

33. Call KM, Glaser T, Ito CY, Buckler AJ, Pelletier J, Haber DA,
Rose EA, Kral A, Yeger H, Lewis WH, Jones C, Housman DE:
Isolation and characterization of a zinc finger polypeptide gene at
the human chromosome 11 Wilms' tumor locus. Cell 1990;
60:509-520.

34. Huff V, Villalba F, Strong LC, Saunders GF: Alteration of the
WT1 gene in patients with Wilms' tumor and genitourinary anomalies. Am J Hum Genet 1991; 49:44.

35. Pelletier J, Bruening W, Kashtan CE, Mauer SM, Manivel JC,
Striegel JE, Houghton DC, Junien C, Habib R, Fouser L, Fine
RN, Silverman BL, Haber DA, Housman D: Germline mutations
in the Wilms' tumor suppressor gene are associated with abnormal
urogenital development in Denys-Drash syndrome. Cell 1991;
67:437-447.

36. Bruening W, Bardeesy N, Silverman BL, Cohn RA, Aronson AJ,
Housman D, Pelletier J: Germline intronic and exonic mutations
in the Wilms' tumor gene (WT1) affecting urogenital development.
Nature Genetics 1992; 1:144-148.

37. Coppes MJ, Liefers GJ, Higuchi M, Zinn AB, Balfe JW, Williams
BRG: Inherited *WT1* mutations in Denys-Drash syndrome. Cancer Res 1992; 52:6125-6128.

38. Ogawa O, Eccles MR, Mueller RF, Holdaway MDD, Reeve AE: A
novel insertional mutation at the third zinc finger coding region of
the WT1 gene in Denys-Drash syndrome. Hum Molec Genet 1993;
2:203-204.

39. Clarkson PA, Davies HL, Williams DM, Chaudhary R, Hughes IA, Patterson MN: Mutational screening of the Wilms' tumor gene, WT1, in males with genital abnormalities. J Med Genet 1993; 30:767-772.

40. Coppes MJ, Huff V, Pelletier J: Denys-Drash syndrome: Relating a clinical disorder to genetic alterations in the tumor suppressor gene *WT1*. J Ped 1993; 123:673-678.

41. Nordenskjöld A, Friedman E, Anvret M: WT1 mutations in patients with Denys-Drash syndrome: A novel mutation in exon 8 and paternal allele origin. Hum Genet 1994; 93:115-120.

42. Sakai A, Tadokoro K, Yanagisawa H, Nagafuchi S, Hoshikawa N, Suzuki T, Kohsaka T, Hasegawa T, Nakahori Y, Yamada M: A novel mutation of the WT1 gene (a tumor suppressor gene for Wilms' tumor) in a patient with Denys-Drash syndrome. Hum Molec Genet 1993; 2:1969-1970.

43. Little MH, Williamson KA, Mannens M, Kelsey A, Gosden C, Hastie ND, van Heyningen V: Evidence that WT1 mutations in Denys-Drash syndrome patients may act in a dominant-negative fashion. Hum Molec Genet 1993; 2:259-264.

44. Pritchard-Jones K, Fleming S, Davidson D, Bickmore W, Porteous D, Gosden C, Bard J, Buckler A, Pelletier J, Housman D, Van Heyningen V, Hastie N: The candidate Wilms' tumour gene is involved in genitourinary development. Nature 1990; 346:194-197.

CHAPTER 8

OTHER LOCI IMPLICATED
IN WILMS TUMOR

INTRODUCTION

There are several features of Wilms tumor and *WT1* mutations that make it clear that the original two-hit hypothesis proposed by Knudson and Strong[1] is inadequate to explain the etiology of this tumor. Although inactivation as proposed in the two-hit hypothesis of the *WT1* gene has indeed been described in certain Wilms tumors (see chapter 7), its incidence (less than 15%) indicates the likely existence of alternative loci involved in the development of this pediatric renal malignancy. Moreover, at least some Wilms tumors are heterozygous for the mutant *WT1* allele: that is, tumor initiation did not require the loss of both wild-type alleles (see chapter 7).

The low frequency of *WT1* mutations reflects, in part at least, the fact that sequencing of the *WT1* gene in tumors has concentrated on the coding regions of the gene. As a result, mutations present in 5' or 3' untranslated regions or within the promoter of *WT1* would not have been detected. Nonetheless, although 15% is probably an underestimate of the frequency of Wilms tumors harboring *WT1* mutations, there are clearly genetic factors other than *WT1* that are important in tumor development.

NEPHROGENIC RESTS, *WT1* MUTATIONS AND WILMS TUMOR

Nephrogenic rests (NR) are foci of undifferentiated renal cells found within the normal kidney tissue of Wilms tumor patients

Wilms Tumor: Clinical and Molecular Characterization, by Max J. Coppes, Christine E. Campbell, and Bryan R.G. Williams. © 1995 R.G. Landes Company.

(see chapter 2). The frequency of NRs is significantly higher than
the frequency of tumors,[2] suggesting that NRs represent premalignant lesions of which only a fraction progress to form a tumor.
Recently, two patients have been described in whom the same
mutation in the *WT1* gene is expressed in both an NR and the
tumor.[3] Thus, mutations in the *WT1* gene may precede the progression from NR to Wilms tumor. In the first case,[3] the *WT1*
mutation was a heterozgyous missense mutation in both the NR
and the tumor. This patient raises the question of whether some
WT1 mutations can act as dominant-negative mutations (see also
chapter 7) and thus exert a phenotypic effect even in the presence
of wild-type protein. One caveat to any discussion of dominant-
negative *WT1* mutations must be kept in mind. Even though transcripts encoding both mutant and wild-type *WT1* alleles are present,
there has been no direct demonstration of coexpression of mutant
and wild-type protein in this or any other tumor. In the second
case,[3] both the tumor and the NR were homozygous for a frameshift mutation that encodes a truncated protein of less than half
the size of the full-length protein. This observation implies that,
while loss of functional WT1 protein may be the initiating event
in the formation of at least a subset of Wilms tumors, additional
changes must occur to progress to a clinically identifiable tumor.

UNDETECTABLE *WT1* MUTATIONS

Our current estimates of the frequency of *WT1* mutations in
Wilms tumors are largely based on sequencing of genomic DNA.
A recent report[4] has suggested that a significant fraction of Wilms
tumors may exhibit a splicing defect in the *WT1* gene that results
in an in-frame deletion of the 123 nucleotides corresponding to
exon 2. The resulting transcript encodes a protein internally deleted for 41 amino acids with respect to wild-type WT1. Although
the deleted transcripts most commonly represented <10% of the
total *WT1* message, the smaller message was not detected in normal human fetal kidney or normal mouse tissues that express *WT1*.
In vitro experiments suggested that the transcriptional regulatory
properties of the deleted protein differ from the wild-type protein.
This was based on the observation that transfection of a construct
directing the synthesis of the deleted protein into a Wilms tumor,
derived cell line RM1 did not result in growth suppression, whereas
transfection of the wild-type construct did. Moreover, in transient

transfection experiments, wild-type *WT1* repressed transcription of an EGR1-CAT chimeric gene approximately 4-fold, while *WT1*-del2 resulted in 2-fold transcriptional activation of the same gene. However, it was not specifically demonstrated that tumor cells actually synthesize the deleted protein. Thus the frequency of exon 2 deletions and their contribution to the etiolgoy of Wilms tumors remains to be determined. Nonetheless, this observation suggests that WT1 function may be altered even in tumors with no apparent mutations within the coding sequence of the *WT1* gene itself. In this case the presumptive mutation could either lie within a non-transcribed region of *WT1* that alters splicing or in the splicing machinery. There may be other Wilms tumors in which similar mutations or alterations have occurred. Because most of the mutation screening that has been carried out on Wilms tumors has involved analysis of DNA not RNA, mutations that delete entire exons would be missed, especially if they represent processing mutations that affect only a small proportion of cellular transcripts. There are currently two assays for functional WT1 protein. The first utilizes truncated recombinant protein and either DNase footprinting, gel mobility shift assays or methylation-protection assays to assay for DNA binding ability. The second assay involves transient transfection of a *WT1* expression construct and a reporter plasmid and measures the ability of the transfected WT1 to activate or repress transcription of the reporter gene which is driven by a promoter that includes a DNA binding site for WT1. There are no assays for endogenous WT1 protein function and thus we have no way of directly assessing whether the protein synthesized by any given tumor is functional within that tumor. This is potentially an important issue as there are several factors that may alter WT1 function (see chapter 6) including posttranscriptional modifications and the presence or absence of interacting proteins.

Another possible source of *WT1* mutations that would not be detected by sequencing genomic DNA is altered gene expression as a result of altered DNA methylation. One report on this subject has suggested that there may be altered DNA methylation in the region of the *WT1* gene based on restriction digests of normal kidney and tumor DNA using NruI and NotI (methylation sensitive enzymes).[5] In general, hypomethylation of a region several hundred kilobases 5' of the *WT1* gene correlated with the degree of *WT1* expression as measured by Northern analysis. Normal human fetal kidney as well as several Wilms tumors that express high levels of *WT1* mRNA were largely unmethylated at a diagnostic NruI site, while the same site was heavily methylated in adult kidney and tumors expressing little or no *WT1*. However, there was at least one exception in which *WT1* expression was high in spite of complete methylation of the NruI site. A second genomic region 3' of *WT1* was hypermethylated in tumors. If site-specific methylation of one *WT1* allele in a heterozygous tumor can lead to loss of expression of that allele, this could result in cells that retain a wild-type *WT1* allele but fail to express transcripts encoding wild-type protein. As most Wilms tumors have been analyzed only at the DNA and not the RNA level, this mechanism of phenotypic expression of a recessive *WT1* mutation would not necesssarily have been detected.

WILMS TUMOR AND *WIT1*

An antisense transcript of *WT1*, named WIT1 (see chapter 4), may also play a role in Wilms tumorigenesis. The *WT1* gene is one of several genes described to date for which the transcription unit includes an antisense transcript. Other examples include the human protooncogene *N-myc*.[6] Thus far, no mutations have been specifically localized in *WIT1* in either Wilms tumors or patients with DDS (see chapter 7), but this gene has not been examined in any great detail. Moreover, because a large open reading frame has not been identified in *WIT1*, it has been difficult to distinguish between possible polymorphisms and mutations (Max J. Coppes, unpublished data). However, some observations suggest that *WIT1* may indeed be involved in Wilms tumorigenesis, either on its own or by regulating *WT1* transcription. First, *WIT1* is subject to differential splicing.[7] Second, at least some of the *WIT1* transcripts are partially complementary to the first exon of *WT1*.[7,8] Third, WIT1 and *WT1* exhibit the same temporal and spacial pattern of expression.[9,10] Finally, the murine *Wt1* locus also appears to contain an antisense transcript (Bryan R.G. Williams, unpublished observations) which has limited sequence homology with human *WIT1*. One possible mechanism whereby *WIT1* might regulate *WT1* is by repressing protein synthesis through the antisense transcripts that include the first exon of *WT1*.[11-13] However, to date, there is no evidence to support this hypothesis.

LOSS OF HETEROZYGOSITY
FOR CHROMOSOME 1p AND 16q

Some of the genetic changes required for the development of Wilms tumor are probably associated with other regions of the human genome that exhibit loss of heterozygosity (LOH) in tumors. In addition to loss of heterozygosity at chromosome 11p found in 40-70% of tumors, LOH studies have also demonstrated a higher-than-expected incidence of 1p (~12%) and 16 q (~17%) loss.[14-16] One study has suggested that 16q loss in particular is associated with a poor prognosis,[16] implying that the putative suppressor gene on 16q is not involved in tumor initiation but rather in tumor progression. A possible candidate gene is the uvomorulin or E-cadherin gene. Uvomorulin is an intracellular adhesion molecule for which downregulated expression is associated with a number of disease states, including prostate carcinoma,[17,18] breast cancer[19-21] and skin cancers.[22] In the mouse, downregulation of this gene is associated with polycystic kidney disease.[23] In the absence of the identification of one or more Wilms tumors carrying mutations within uvomorulin however, the identity of the 16q Wilms tumor progression gene remains unresolved and other candidate genes are likely to be identified as mapping of the long arm of chromosome 16 proceeds.

WILMS TUMOR AND BECKWITH-WIEDEMANN
SYNDROME

As mentioned in chapter 3, LOH at the *WT1* locus is frequently accompanied by a similar loss of heterozygosity for all genes distal to *WT1* on chromosome 11. Since there appears to be a second Wilms tumor locus at 11p15, this can make it difficult to separate the contributions to tumor phenotype of changes at the *WT1* locus from changes at the second 11p locus. The existence of a Wilms tumor predisposing gene mapping to chromosomal region 11p15.5 has been inferred from two observations (see also chapter 3). The first is that, although most tumors that exhibit LOH for 11p13 are also homozygous for 11p15 since 11p15 is distal to 11p13 (see Fig. 8.1), there is a subset of sporadic Wilms tumors that exhibit LOH at 11p15 but not 11p13.[15,24-27] The second observation is that the inherited genetic disorder Beckwith-Wiedemann syndrome (BWS, see chapter 1) which maps to 11p15.5 is associated with an increased incidence of several embryonal tumors, most notably Wilms tumor.[28,29] The frequency of this tumor among patients with BWS is ~5%.[30] However, unlike the WAGR syndrome, which is associated exclusively with an increased incidence of Wilms tumor, patients with BWS also exhibit a higher than expected frequency of hepatoblastomas, rhabdomyo-sarcomas and

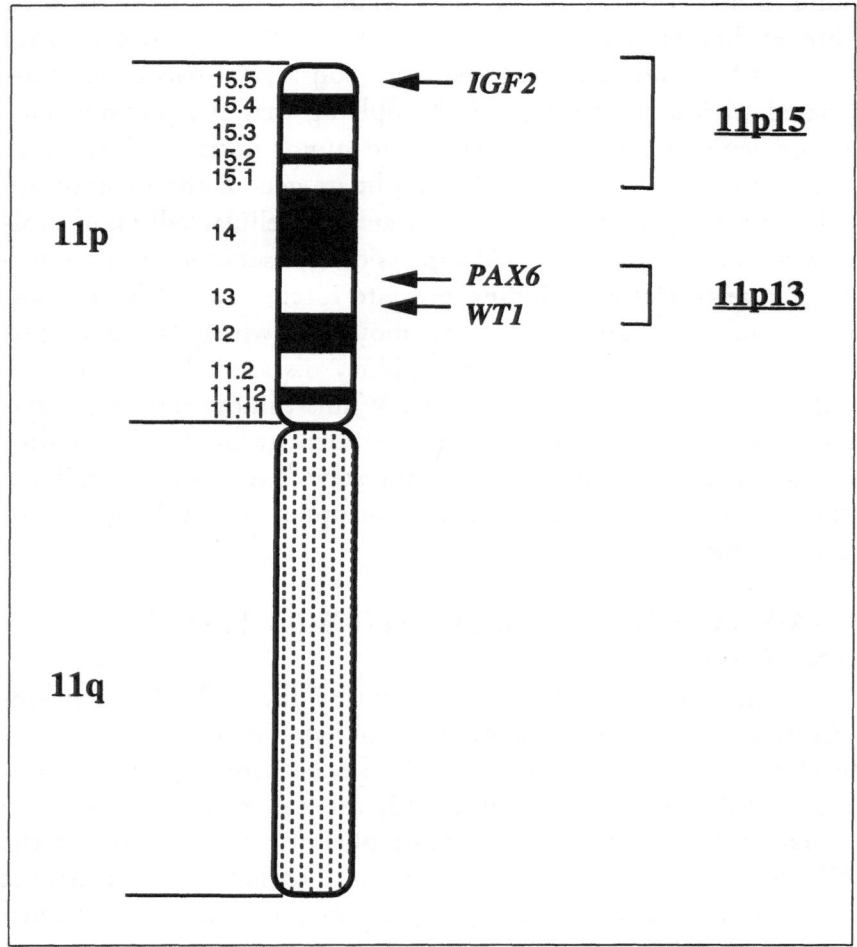

Fig. 8.1. Chromosome 11. Diagrammatic representation of the chromosomal location of the Wilms tumor suppressor gene WT1, the aniridia gene PAX6 (both at chromosome 11p13), and the IGF2 gene on chromosome 11p15.5. The Wilms tumor suppressor gene at chromosome 11p15 and the Beckwith-Wiedemann gene have not identified. Children with the WAGR syndrome have a deletion involving 11p13, while virtually all children with the Denys-Drash syndrome carry a constitutional point mutation of the WT1 gene. Reprinted with permission from M.J. Coppes et al, Genetic events in the development of Wilms' tumor, New England Journal of Medicine 1994; 331:586-590, Copyright © Massachusetts Medical Society.

adrenocorticocarcinomas. There is also evidence suggesting that LOH at 11p15 is associated with perilobar nephrogenic rests and a later age of onset of disease while LOH at 11p13 or *WT1* mutations (i.e. in patients with DDS) are associated with intralobar nephrogeneic rests and an earlier age of onset.[31,32] Based on the developmental pattern exhibited by the kidney, with maturation proceeding from the medulla to the cortex, this observation might suggest that the Wilms tumor gene mapping to 11p15 plays a role later in development than the 11p13 gene and might even be a target of regulation by *WT1*, through the ability of *WT1* to act as a transcriptional regulator of other genes. Alternatively, the report of a Wilms tumor patient who exhibited LOH for most of 11p but was heterozygous for a *WT1* mutation, raises the possibility that the WT1 protein may be involved in protein-protein interactions with a protein encoded by a gene mapping to 11p15. There is no direct evidence to support either of these hypotheses. This issue will only be resolved following the identification and cloning of *WT2*, the Wilms tumor suppressor gene at chromosome 11p15.

The association of BWS with an increased incidence of Wilms tumors suggests that there may be a single gene, *WT2* involved in both BWS and some of the sporadic Wilms tumors that exhibit LOH for 11p15. Alternatively, each disorder may be caused by distinct but neighboring genes. There are several aspects of BWS however which raise the possibility that identifying the appropriate gene(s) may not be straightforward. First, BWS shows a very high frequency of discordance amongst monozygotic twins, suggesting that expression may be affected by epigenetic events in addition to classical mutations. Second, the cytogenetic anomalies associated with BWS are primarily translocations and duplications, rather than deletions as one might expect for a tumor suppressor gene. These observations suggest that the Wilms tumor predisposing gene at 11p15 exerts its effects through overexpression rather than loss of expression of a functional gene product. Genetic changes resulting in overexpression of a gene product are likely to be more difficult to detect than diminished expression following gene deletions, frameshift and missense mutations, such as the ones that have been described for *WT1* (see chapter 7) As a further complication, the translocations associated with BWS map to two discrete regions of 11p15, separated by greater than 10 Mb (Fig. 8.2). This observation raises the possibility that there is more than one BWS gene, or alternatively, that disruption of the normal chromosome sequence through translocation or duplication has long-range effects on the expression of genes many megabases from the site of the translocation or duplication. The pattern of inheritance of BWS is also suggestive of an imprinted gene. Imprinting and its possible role in Wilms tumor is discussed in more detail below.

WILMS TUMOR AND PERLMAN SYNDROME

Another syndrome associated with a significant incidence of Wilms tumor is Perlman syndrome. This is a relatively rare autosomal recessive condition with characteristic facial features, a high neonatal mortality rate, mental retardation and kidney abnormalities including Wilms tumor. Given the rarity of the disease, it is difficult to acertain the frequency of Wilms tumor but, to date, every patient (5/5) has either developed Wilms tumor or shown indications of small tumors upon autopsy.[33] It is worth noting that in at least one patient, DNA from the Wilms tumor exhibited LOH of 11p15 markers. The prevailing opinion appears to be that this syndrome is distinct from BWS but also maps to 11p15. Recently two patients with Perlman syndrome have been described who carry a constitutional deletion of 11p15 that does not include 16F2 (John Cowell, personal communication, see Fig. 8.2). This deletion may define the location of the *WT2* gene. Alternatively, the deletion may affect IGF2 expression through a long range perturbation of gene expression. This issue remains to be resolved.

IMPRINTING, *IGF2, H19* AND WILMS TUMOR

One intriguing facet of the involvement of a gene or genes at 11p15 in the etiology of Wilms tumor is the existence of several candidate genes already cloned from this chromosomal region (Fig. 8.2). The most interesting with respect to Wilms tumor are *IGF2* and *H19*. IGF2, or insulin-like growth factor II, is a growth factor highly expressed during the embryonic development of many organs, including the kidney. *IGF2* gene expression is increased in Wilms tumors[34] but it was initially unclear whether this represented aberrant regulation of transcription or was merely a reflection of the tumor consisting of cells in an embryonic stage of kidney development. However, *IGF2* is now known to be one of at least seven genes that have been shown to be subject to genomic im-

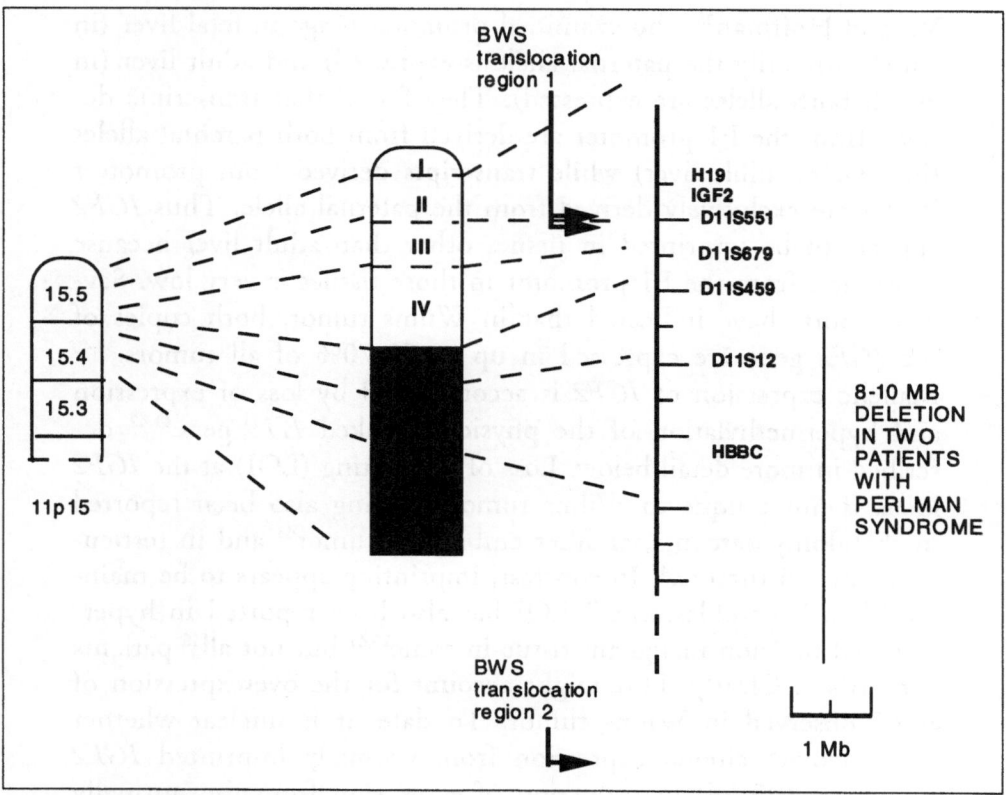

Fig. 8.2. Map of human chromosome 11p15. This map indicates the approximate locations of the two BWS translocation regions, H19, IGF2 and the region heterozygously deleted in two Perlman patients (John Cowell, personal communication)

printing in either or both mice and humans. All autosomal genes are present in two copies in mammalian cells, one allele derived from the female gamete and one from the male. Imprinting, in this context, refers to genes which are differentially expressed depending upon whether they are maternal or paternal in origin. For *IGF2*, in most tissues including fetal kidney, only the paternally inherited allele is normally expressed.[35,36] In humans both IGF2 alleles are expressed in adult liver[37] while in mice imprinting is lost in the choroid plexus and leptomeninges at mid-gestation.[35] In human liver where *IGF2* is biallelically expressed, expression is predominantly from one of the four *IGF2* promoters (the P1 promoter), suggesting that imprinting is not only gene specific but may be promoter specific. This has recently been confirmed by

Vu and Hoffman[38] who examined promoter usage in fetal liver (in which primarily the paternal allele is expressed) and adult liver (in which both alleles are expressed). They found that transcripts derived from the P1 promoter are derived from both parental alleles (in fetal or adult liver) while transcripts derived from promoters P2-P4 are exclusively derived from the paternal allele. Thus *IGF2* appears to be imprinted in tissues other than adult liver because expression from the P1 promotor in those tissues is very low. Several reports have indicated that in Wilms tumor, both copies of the *IGF2* gene are expressed in up to 50-70% of all tumors.[39,40] Biallelic expression of *IGF2* is accompanied by loss of expression and hypermethylation of the physically linked *H19* gene[41,42] described in more detail below. Loss of imprinting (LOI) at the *IGF2* locus is not unique to Wilms tumors, having also been reported in rhabdomyosarcoma, another embryonal tumor[43] and in testicular germ cell tumors.[44] In contrast, imprinting appears to be maintained in hepatoblastoma.[45] LOI has also been reported in hypertrophied but non-malignant tissue in some[29,41] but not all[46] patients with BWS. Clearly, LOI might account for the overexpression of *IGF2* observed in Wilms tumor. To date, it is unclear whether LOI involves altered expression from normally imprinted *IGF2* promoters (P2-P4) or induction of expression from the normally liver specific and biallellically expressed P1 promoter.

It is worth noting that in Wilms tumors exhibiting LOH for 11p15, it is always the maternally derived chromosome that is lost.[15] LOH rarely involves total chromosome loss but rather results from either mitotic recombination or chromosomal non-disjunction such that the maternally derived material that is lost is replaced with paternally derived chromosomal material (Fig. 8.3). Either of these events will result in two active paternal *IGF2* alleles and might again explain the overexpression of *IGF2* mRNA observed in many tumors. Recently it has been shown that a loss of IGF2 function, achieved through a transgenic mouse knockout, results in a significantly reduced rate of pancreatic tumor growth when knockout mice are crossed into a background of increased pancreatic tumors.[47] Transgenic mice overexpressing IGF2 on the other hand exhibit an increased incidence of several different malignancies.[48] These observations suggest that overexpression of IGF2, while it might not initiate the malignant process, may promote tumor growth or perhaps increase the number of target cells and there-

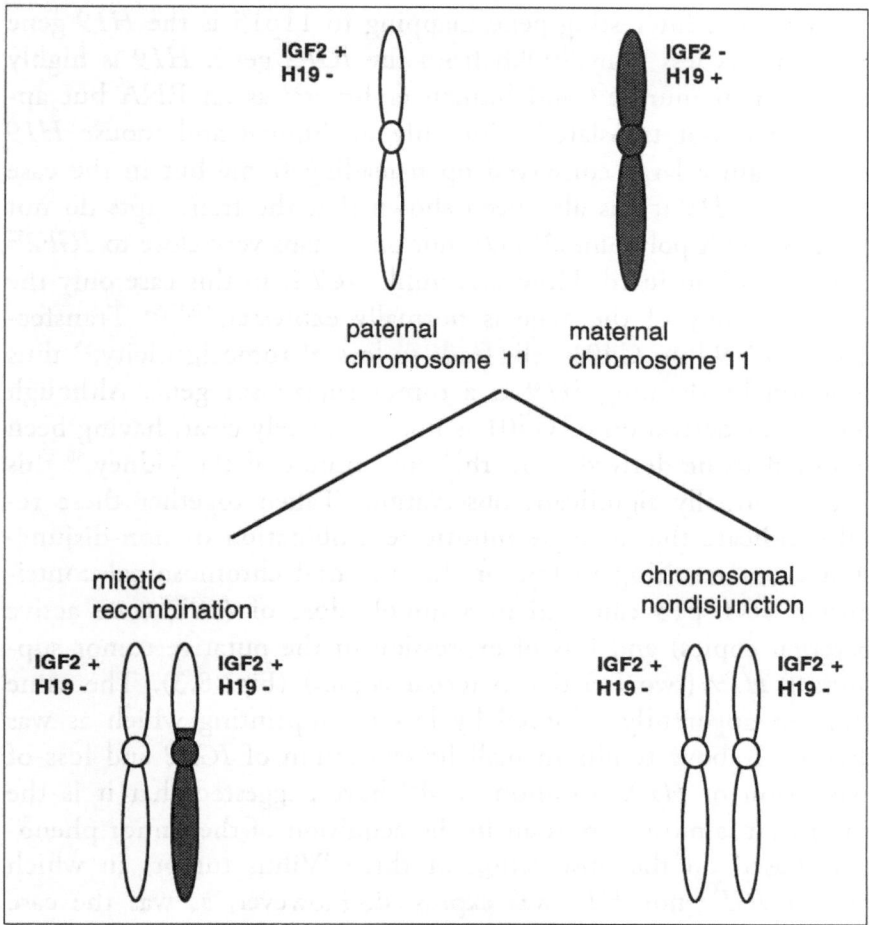

Fig. 8.3. *Mitotic recombination or chromosome non-disjunction involving IGF2 and H19. Because IGF2 and H19 are closely linked and are imprinted in opposite directions, a single mitotic recombination or chromosomal nondisjunction event will result in a cell that has two copies of paternally derived 11p material and thus overexpresses the former and underexpresses the latter. In theory, either mitotic recombination or chromosomal nondisjunction should be reciprocal events : that is for every cell produced that has two copies of paternal chromosome material there should be a cell with two maternal copies of the same material, i.e., overexpressing H19 and underexpressing IGF2. The fact that we do not observe such cells suggests either that their phenotype is normal and therefore indistinguishable from the majority of cells of individual or that such cells die and are never detected.*

fore the probability that one of them will suffer a tumor initiating event. One significant difference between patients with BWS and transgenic mice overexpressing the *IGF2* gene is that the former develop pediatric malignancies while the latter develop tumors only after a long latency period.[48]

A second interesting gene mapping to 11p15 is the *H19* gene which maps less than 200kb from the *IGF2* gene. *H19* is highly expressed in murine[49] and human embryos[50] as an RNA but apparently is not translated. Not only do human and mouse *H19* not contain a large conserved open reading frame but in the case of mouse *H19* it has also been shown that the transcripts do not associate with polysomes.[51] *H19* not only maps very close to *IGF2*[52] but is also imprinted. However, unlike *IGF2*, in this case only the maternal copy of the gene is normally expressed.[50,53,54] Transfection of *H19* into G401 cells leads to loss of tumorigenicity,[55] thus functionally defining *H19* as a tumor suppressor gene. Although the tumor derivation of G401 is not completely clear, having been reported to be derived from rhabdoid tumor of the kidney,[56] this is a potentially significant observation. Taken together these results indicate that a single mitotic recombination or non-disjunction event resulting in loss of the maternal chromosomal contribution at 11p15 can lead to a double dose of *IGF2* (two active paternal copies) and loss of expression of the putative tumor suppressor *H19* (two inactive paternal copies) (Fig. 8.3). The same effect is apparently achieved by loss of imprinting which as was described above results in biallelic expression of *IGF2* and loss of expression of *H19*. Moulton et al[42] have suggested that it is the latter that is most important in the acquision of the tumor phenotype based on the observation of three Wilms tumors in which neither *IGF2* nor *H19* was expressed. However, as was the case with the presence of *WT1* mutations in premalignant nephrogenic rests, loss or reduction of *H19* expression has also been observed in the normal kidney of Wilms tumor patients.[42] This observation implies that if loss of *H19* expression serves as an initiating event for tumorigenesis, additional events are required to generate a clinically detectable tumor. Moreover, if loss of *H19* expression is primarily acquired through events other than classical mutations, such as loss of heterozygosity or alterations in methylation status of the DNA which affect more than one gene at a time, it may be difficult to prove that *H19* is serving as a tumor suppressor gene for Wilms tumor initiation. Therefore, it remains to be seen whether either *IGF2* or *H19* is the putative Wilms tumor gene *WT2* at 11p15 or whether there is yet another tumor suppressor mapping to this chromosomal location, possibly localized to the deletion associated with Perlman syndrome (see above).

It should be noted that LOH at 11p15 occurs in a number of sporadic tumors in addition to Wilms tumors, including other pediatric tumors associated with BWS such as rhabdomyosarcoma and hepatoblastoma,[57] as well as in some adult tumors such as breast, ovarian and non-small cell lung carcinoma.[58]

WT1 itself is not subjected to imprinting at least in the kidney.[59] There has been a recent report that the paternally-derived *WT1* allele is frequently silent in the placenta and brain[60] but while this might affect some functions of *WT1*, it is unlikely to contribute to its role in nephrogenesis or the development of Wilms tumor.

WILMS TUMOR AND LI-FRAUMENI SYNDROME

Li-Fraumeni syndrome is a cancer predisposition syndrome associated with mutations in the *p53* tumor suppressor gene.[61] Individuals heterozygous for *p53* mutations are at increased risk for a number of different tumors including osteosarcoma, adrenal cortical carcinoma and early onset breast cancer. In addition, there are numerous sporadic tumors such as colon carcimoma and glioblastoma which also exhibit a high incidence of mutations in *p53*.[62] The suggestion has been made that Wilms tumor might be a rare component of the Li-Fraumeni syndrome based on a study of the family histories of 176 children with Wilms tumor.[63] However, given the rarity of Li-Fraumeni syndrome and the relatively high frequency of Wilms tumor, this observation may represent sampling error and not be biologically significant. Moreover, the incidence of *p53* mutations in sporadic Wilms tumors unlike that observed in many other malignancies is relatively low (probably less than 10%).[64,65] However, it has been suggested that Wilms tumors carrying *p53* mutations may phenotypically be different from those Wilms tumor not carrying a *p53* mutation.[66] This hypothesis, in conjunction with a report that *WT1* and *p53* may engage in protein-protein interactions that affect the transcriptional regulatory functions of both proteins (see chapter 6), suggests the role of *p53* in Wilms tumor merits further investigation.

FAMILIAL WILMS TUMOR

In addition to the genes described above, there is at least one additional Wilms tumor predisposing gene associated with familial Wilms tumor. Because this is a rare disorder accounting for less than 3% of all Wilms tumors, it is difficult to know whether there is more than one gene associated with familial Wilms. However, analysis of several large pedigrees have excluded both 11p and 16q as the map location of the predisposing gene in these families.[67-70] Once this gene or genes are cloned it will obviously be important to test their involvement in sporadic Wilms tumors.

WILMS TUMOR AND OTHER DISEASE ASSOCIATIONS

In addition to its association with WAGR syndrome, DDS, BWS and Perlman syndrome there have been rare reports of individuals afflicted with Wilms tumor in conjunction with another genetic disorder. For example, a patient with type I neurofibromatosis and Wilms tumor has been described[71] as has a patient with Prader-Willi syndrome and Wilms tumor.[72] Although it is likely that Wilms tumor in these patients is simply a coincidence it remains possible that rare alleles of genes involved in neurofibromatosis or Prader-Willi may also initiate or promote Wilms tumor development.

CONCLUSION

Although mutations in the *WT1* gene at chromosome 11p13 clearly play a role in the initiation of certain Wilms tumors, the biology of this cancer is complex. There is genetic evidence for at least two other genes that probably play a role in tumor inititiation (the gene or genes at 11p15 and the gene or genes associated with familial Wilms tumor). In addition the tumor suppressor *p53* and unidentified genes on 16q and 1p probably play roles in tumor progression. Moreover, it is apparent based on the presence of *WT1* mutations in nephrogenic rests and in patients with DDS that even when a mutation in *WT1* occurs, other events are necessary to lead to the development of a tumor. To further complicate the picture, epigenetic events such as imprinting and DNA methylation are probably also important in the etiology of this cancer.

REFERENCES

1. Knudson AG, Strong LC: Mutation and cancer: A model for Wilms' tumor of kidney. J Natl Cancer Inst 1972; 48:313-324.
2. Beckwith JB: Precursor lesions of Wilms tumor: clinical and biological implications. Med Pediatr Oncol 1993; 21:158-168.
3. Park S, Bernard A, Bove KE, Sens DA, Hazen-Martin DJ, Garvin HA, Haber DA: Inactivation of *WT1* in nephrogenic rests, genetic precursors to Wilms' tumour. Nature Genetics 1993; 5:363-367.

4. Haber DA, Park S, Maheswaran S, Englert C, Re GG, Hazen-Martin DJ, Sens DA, Garvin AJ: WT-1-mediated growth suppression of Wilms tumor cells expressing *WT1* splicing variant. Science 1993; 262:2057-2059.

5. Royer PB, Schneider S: Wilms' tumor-specific methylation pattern in 11p13 detected by PFGE. Genes Chromo Cancer 1992; 5:132-140.

6. Armstrong BC, Krystal GW: Isolation and characterization of complementary DNA from N-cym, a gene encoded by the DNA strand opposite to N-myc. Cell Growth Diff 1992; 3:385-390.

7. Campbell CE, Huang A, Gurney AL, Kessler PM, Hewitt JA, Williams BRG: Antisense transcripts and protein binding motifs within the Wilms tumour (WT1) locus. Oncogene 1994; 9:583-595.

8. Eccles MR, Grubb G, Ogawa O, Szeto J, Reeve AE: Cloning of novel Wilms tumor gene (WT1) cDNAs: evidence for antisense transcription of WT1. Oncogene 1994; 9:2059-2063.

9. Huang A, Campbell CE, Bonetta L, McAndrews -Hill M, Chilton-MacNeill S, Coppes MJ, Law DJ, Feinberg AP, Yeger H, Williams BRG: Tissue, developmental, and tumor-specific expression of divergent transcripts in Wilms tumor. Science 1990; 250:991-994.

10. Yeger H, Cullinane C, Flenniken A, Chilton-MacNeill S, Campbell C, Huang A, Bonetta L, Coppes MJ, Thorner P, Williams BRG: Coordinate expression of Wilms tumor genes correlates with Wilms tumor phenotypes. Cell Growth Differentiation 1992; 3:855-864.

11. Kimelmann D: Regulation of eukaryotic gene expression by natural antisense transcripts - the case of the modifying reaction. Gene Regulation 1992; 1:1-10.

12. Liebhaber SA, Russell JE, Cash FE, Eshleman SS: Inhibition of messenger RNA translation by antisense sequences. Gene Regulation 1992; 1:163-174.

13. Silverman TA, Noguchi M, Safer B: Corrdinate expression of Wilms tumor genes correlates with Wilms tumor phenotypes. Cell Growth Differentiation 1992; 3:855-864.

14. Maw MA, Grundy PE, Millow LJ, Eccles MR, Dunn RS, Smith PJ, Feinberg AP, Law DJ, Paterson MC, Telzerow PE, Callen DF, Thompson AD, Richards RI, Reeve AE: A third Wilms' tumor locus on chromosome 16q. Cancer Res 1992; 52:3094-3098.

15. Coppes MJ, Bonetta L, Huang A, Hoban P, Chilton-MacNeill S, Campbell CE, Weksberg R, Yeger H, Reeve AE, Williams BRG: Loss of heterozygosity mapping in Wilms tumor indicates the involvement of three distinct regions and a limited role for non-disjunction or mitotic recombination. Genes Chrom Cancer 1992; 5:326-334.

16. Grundy PE, Telzerow PE, Breslow N, Moskess J, Huff V, Paterson MC: Loss of heterozygosity for chromosomes 16q and 1p in Wilms' tumors predicts an adverse outcome. Cancer Res 1994; 54:2331-2333.

17. Bussemakers JJG, Vanmoorselaar RJA, Giroldi LA, Ichikawa T, Isaacs JT, Takeichi M, Debruyne FJ, Schalken JA: Decreased expression of E-cadherin in the progression of rat prostatic cancer. Cancer Res 1992; 52:2916-2922.

18. Umbas R, Schalken JA, Aalders TW, Carter BS, Karthaus HFM, Schaafsma HE, Debruyne FMJ, Isaacs WB: Expression of the cellular adhesion molecule E-caherin is reduced or absent in high-grade prostate cancer. Cancer Res 1992; 52:5104-5109.

19. Sommers CL, E. HS, Skerker JM, Worland P, Torri JA, Thompson EW, Byers SW, Gelmann EP: Loss of epithelial markers and acquisition of vimentin expression in adriamycin-resistant and vinblastine-resistant human breast cancer cell lines. Cancer Res 1992; 52:5190-5197.

20. Inoue M, Ogawa H, Miyata M, Shiozaki H, Tanizawa O: Expression of E-cadherin in normal, benign, and malignant tissues of female genital organs. Am J Clin Pathol 1992; 98:76-80.

21. Behrens J: The role of cell adhesion molecules in cancer invasion and metastasis. Breast Cancer Res Treat 1993; 24:175-184.

22. Ruggeri B, Caamano J, Slaga TJ, Conti CJ, Nelson WJ, Kleinszanto AJP: Alterations in the expression of uvomorulin and Na+, K+ - adenosine triphosphatase during mouse skin tumor progression. Am J Pathol 1992; 140:1179-1185.

23. Rocco MV, Neilson EG, Hoyer JR, Ziyadeh FN: Attenuated expression of epithelial cell adhesion molecules in murine polycystic kidney disease. Am J Physiol 1992; 262:F679-F686.

24. Jeanpierre C, Antignac C, Beroud C, Lavedan C, Henry I, Saunders G, Williams B, Glaser T, Junien C: Constitutional and somatic deletions of two different regions of maternal chromosome 11 in Wilms tumor. Genomics 1990; 7:434-438.

25. Baird P, Wadey R, Cowell J: Loss of heterozygosity for chromosome region 11p15 in Wilms tumours is not related to HRAS gene transforming mutations. Oncogene 1991; 6:1147-1149.

26. Chao LY, Huff G, Tomlinson G, Riccardi VM, Strong LC, Saunders GF: Genetic mosaicism in normal tissues of Wilms tumor patients. Nature Genetics 1993; 3:127-131.

27. Gerald WL: The molecular genetics of Wilms tumor: a paradigm of heterogeneity in tumor development. Cancer Investigation 1994; 12:350-359.

28. Schneid H, Vazquez MP, Seurin D, le BY: Loss of heterozygosity in non-tumoral tissue in two children with Beckwith-Wiedemann syndrome. Growth Regulation 1991; 1:168-170.

29. Weksberg R, Shen DR, Fei YL, Song QL, Squire J: Disruption of insulin-like growth factor 2 imprinting in Beckwith-Wiedemann syndrome. Nat Genet 1993; 5:143-150.

30. Wiedemann H-R: Tumours and hemihypertrophy associated with Wiedemann-Beckwith syndrome. Eur J Pediatr 1983; 141:129.

31. Beckwith JB, Kiviat NB, Bonadio JF: Nephrogenic rests, nephroblastomatosis, and the pathogenesis of Wilms' tumor. Pediatr Pathol 1990; 10:1-36.

32. Heppe RK, Koyle MA, Beckwith JB: Nephrogenic rests in Wilms tumor patients with the Drash syndrome. J Urol 1991; 145: 1225-1228.

33. Grundy RG, Pritchard J, Baraitser M, Risdon A, Robards M: Perlman and Wiedemann-Beckwith syndromes: two distinct conditions associated with Wilms tumor. Eur J Pediatr 1992; 151: 895-898.

34. Reeve AE, Eccles MR, Wilkins RJ, Bell GI, Millow LJ: Expression of insulin-like growth factor-II transcripts in Wilms tumor. Nature 1985; 317:258-260.

35. DeChiara TM, Robertson EJ, Efstratiadias A: Parental imprinting of the mouse insulin-like growth factor II gene. Cell 1991; 64:849-859.

36. Giannoukakis N, Deal C, Paquette J, Goodyer CG, Polychronakos C: Parental genomic imprinting of the human IGF-2 gene. Nature Genetics 1993; 4:98-101.

37. Davies SM: Developmental regulation of genomic imprinting of the IGF2 gene in human liver. Cancer Res 1994; 54:2560-2562.

38. Vu TH, Hoffman AR: Promoter-specific imprinting of the human insulin-like growth factor-II gene. Nature 1994; 371:714-717.

39. Ogawa O, Eccles MR, Szeto J, McNoe LA, Yun K, Maw MA, Smith PJ, Reeve AE: Relaxation of Insulin-like Growth factor II gene imprinting implicated in Wilms tumour. Nature 1993; 362:749-751.

40. Rainier S, Johnson LA, Dobry CJ, Ping AJ, Grundy PE, Feinberg AP: Relaxation of imprinted genes in human cancer. Nature 1993; 362:747-749.

41. Steenman MJC, Rainier S, Dobry CJ, Grundy P, Horon IL, Feinberg AP: Loss of imprinting of IGF2 is linked to reduced expression and abnormal methylation of H19 in Wilms tumour. Nature Genetics 1994; 7:433-439.

42. Moulton T, Crenshaw T, Hao Y, Moosikasuwan J, Lin N, Dembitzer F, Hensle T, Weiss L, McMorrow L, Loew T, Kraus W, W. G, Tycko B: Epigenetic lesions at the H19 locus in Wilms tumour patients. Nature Genetics 1994; 7:440-447.

43. Zhan S, Shapiro DN, Helman LJ: Activation of an imprinted allele of the insulin-like growth factor II gene implicated in rhabdomyosarcoma. J Clin Invest 1994; 94:445-448.

44. Van Gurp RJ, Oosterhuis JW, Kalscheuer V, Mariman EC, Looijenga LH: Biallelic expression of the H19 and IGF2 genes in human testicular germ cell tumors. J Natl Cancer Inst 1994; 86:1071-1075.

45. Davies SM: Maintenance of genomic imprinting at the IGF2 locus in hepatoblastoma. Cancer Res 1993; 53:4781-4783.

46. Ohlsson R, Nystrom A, Pfeifer OS, Tohonen V, Hedborg F, Schofield P, Flam F, Ekstrom TJ: IGF2 is parentally imprinted during human embryogenesis and in the Beckwith-Wiedemann syndrome. Nature Genetics 1993; 4:94-97.

47. Christofori G, Naik P, Hanahan D: A second signal supplied by insulin-like growth factor II in oncogene-induced tumorigenesis. Nature 1994; 369:414-418.

48. Rogler CE, Yang D, Rossetti L, Donohoe J, Alt E, Chang CJ, Rosenfeld R, Nelly K, Hintz R: Altered body compostion and increased frequency of diverse malignancies in insulin-like growth factor-II transgenic mice. J Biol Chem 1994; 269:13779-13784.

49. Poirier F, Chan CT, Timmons PM, Robertson EJ, Evans MJ, Rigby PW: The murine H19 gene is activated during embroyonic stem cell differentiation in vitro and at the time of implantation in the developing embryo. Development 1991; 113:1105-1114.

50. Zhang Y, Tycko B: Monoallelic expression of the human *H19* gene. Nature Genetics 1992; 1:40-44.

51. Brannan CI, Dees EC, Ingram RS, Tilghman SM: The product of the H19 gene may function as an RNA. Mol Cell Biol 1990; 10:28-36.

52. Zemel S, Bartolomei MS, Tilghman SM: Physical linkage of 2 mammalian imprinted genes, H19 and insulin-like growth factor-2. Nat Genet 1992; 2:61-65.

53. Bartolomei MS, Zemel S, Tilghman S: Parental imprinting of the mouse H19 gene. Nature 1991; 351:153-155.

54. Rachmilewitz J, Goshen R, Ariel I, Schneider T, de GN, Hochberg A: Parental imprinting of the human H19 gene. Febs Letters 1992; 309:25-28.

55. Hao Y, Crenshaw T, Moulton T, Newcomb E, Tycko B: Tumoursuppressor activity of *H19* RNA. Nature 1993; 365:764-767.

56. Garvin AJ, Re GG, Tarnowski BI, Hazan-Martin DJ, Sens DA: The G401 cell line, utilized for studies of chromosomal changes in Wilms tumor, is derived from a rhabdoid tumor of the kidney. Am J Pathol 1993; 142:375-380.

57. Byrne JA, Simms LA, Little MH, Algar EM, Smith PJ: Three nonoverlapping regions of chromosome arm 11p allele loss identified in infantile tumors of adrenal and liver. Genes Chromosomes Cancer 1993; 8:104-111.

58. Bepler G, Garcia-Blanco MA: Three tumor-suppressor regions on chromsome 11p identified by high-resolution deletion mapping in human non-small-cell lung cancer. Proc Natl Acad Sci USA 1994; 91:5513-5517.

59. Little MH, Dunn R, Byrne JA, Seawright A, Smith PJ, Pritchard JK, van HV, Hastie ND: Equivalent expression of paternally and maternally inherited WT1 alleles in normal fetal tissue and Wilms' tumours. Oncogene 1992; 7:635-641.

60. Jinno Y, Yun K, Hishiwaki K, Kubota T, Ogawa O, Reeve AE, Hiikawa N: Mosaic and polymorphic imprinting of the WT1 gene in humans. Nature Genetics 1994; 6:305-309.

61. Malkin D: P53 and the Li-Fraumeni syndrome. Cancer Genet Cytogenet 1993; 66:83-92.

62. Hinds PW, Weinberg RA: Tumor suppressor genes. Current Opinion in Genet Development 1994; 4:135-141.

63. Hartley AL, Birch JM, Tricker K, Wallace SA, Kelsey AM, Harris M, Jones PH: Wilms tumor in the Li-Fraumeni cancer family syndrome. Cancer Genet Cytogenet 1993; 67:133-135.

64. Waber PG, Chen J, Nisen PD: Infrequency of ras, p53, WT1, or RB gene alternations in Wilms tumors. Cancer 1993; 72:3732-3738.

65. Malkin D, Sexsmith E, Yeger H, Williams BRG, Coppes MJ: Mutations of the *p53* tumor suppressor gene occur infrequently in Wilms tumor. Cancer Res 1994; 54:2077-2079.

66. Bardeesy N, falkoff D, Petruzii M-J, Nowak N, Zabel B, Adam M, Aguiar MC, Grundy P, Shows T, Pelletier J: Anaplastic Wilms' tumour, a subtype displaying poor prognosis, harbours p53 gene mutations. Nature Genetics 1994; 7:91-97.

67. Grundy P, Koufos A, Morgan K, Li FP, Meadows AT, Cavenee WK: Familial predisposition to Wilms' tumour does not map to the short arm of chromosome 11. Nature 1988; 336:374-376.

68. Huff V, Compton DA, Chao LY, Strong LC, Geiser CF, Saunders GF: Lack of linkage of familial Wilms' tumour to chromosomal band 11p13. Nature 1988; 336:377-378.

69. Schwartz CE, Haber DA, Stanton VP, Strong LC, Skolnick MH, Housman DE: Familial predisposition to Wilms tumor does not segregate with the WT1 gene. Genomics 1991; 10:927-30.

70. Huff V, Reeve AE, Leppert M, Strong LC, Douglass EC, Geiser CF, Li FP, Meadows A, Callen DF, Lenoir G, Saunders GF: Nonlinkage of 16q markers to familial predisposition to Wilms tumor. Cancer Res 1992; 52:6117-6120.

71. Perilongo G, Felix CA, Meadows AT, Nowell P, Biegel J, Lange BJ: Sequential development of Wilms tumor, T-cell acute lymphoblastic leukemia, medulloblastoma and myeloid leukemia in a child with type 1 neurofibromatosis: a clinical and cytogenetic case report. Leukemia 1993; 7:912-915.

72. Coppes MJ, Sohl H, Teshima IE, Ledbetter DH, Weksberg R: Wilms tumor in a patient with Prader-Willi syndrome. J Pediatr 1993; 122:730-733.

INDEX

MOLECULAR BIOLOGY
INTELLIGENCE UNIT
AVAILABLE AND UPCOMING TITLES

NEUROSCIENCE INTELLIGENCE UNIT

AVAILABLE AND UPCOMING TITLES

MEDICAL INTELLIGENCE UNIT

AVAILABLE AND UPCOMING TITLES

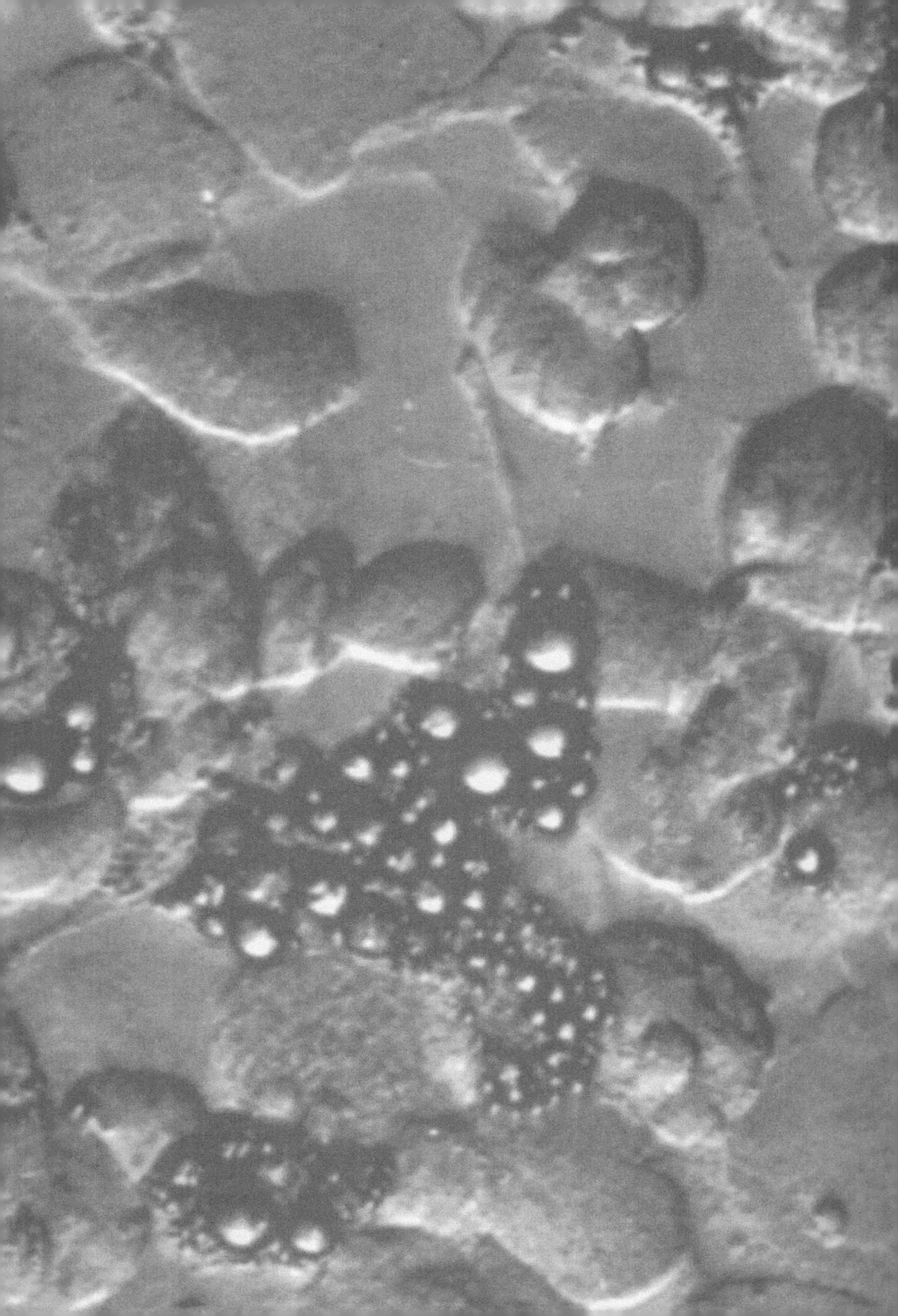

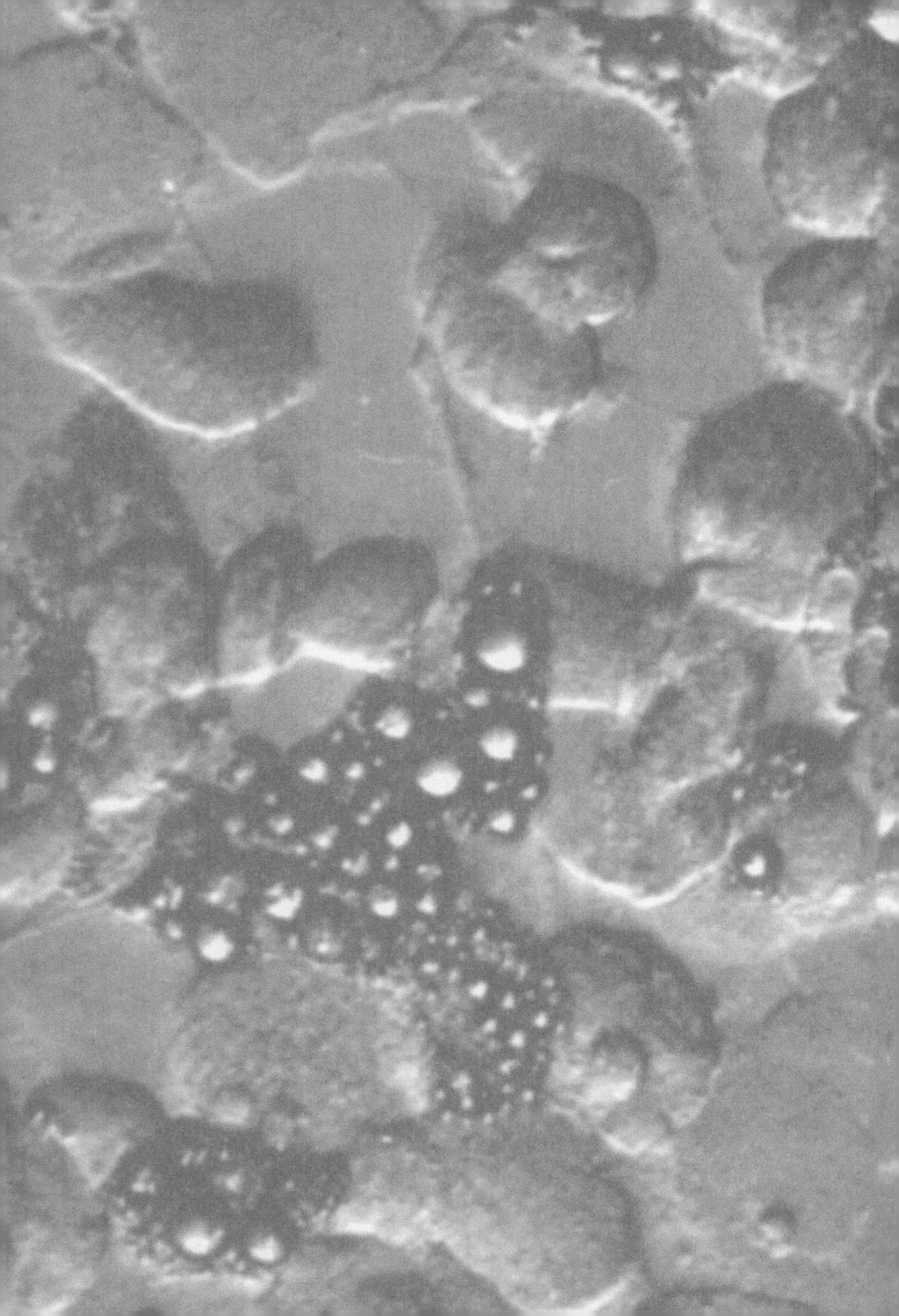